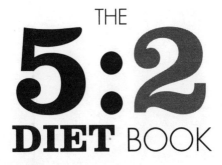

THE

5:2

DIET BOOK

THE 5:2 DIET BOOK

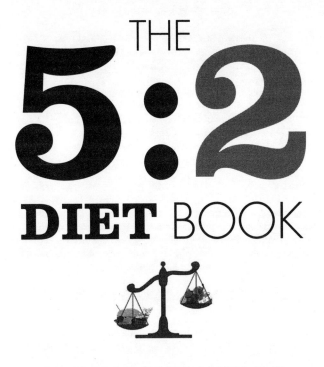

*FEAST FOR 5 DAYS A WEEK AND
FAST FOR JUST 2 TO LOSE WEIGHT,
BOOST YOUR BRAIN AND
TRANSFORM YOUR HEALTH*

KATE HARRISON

This edition first published in Great Britain in 2013 by
Orion Books
an imprint of the Orion Publishing Group Ltd
Orion House, 5 Upper St Martin's Lane,
London WC2H 9EA
An Hachette UK Company

24

A CIP catalogue record for this book is available
from the British Library.

ISBN: 978 1 4091 4669 8
Printed in Great Britain by CPI Group (UK) Ltd, Croydon, CR0 4YY

The Orion Publishing Group's policy is to use papers that are natural, renewable
and recyclable and made from wood grown in sustainable forests. The logging and
manufacturing processes are expected to conform to the environmental regulations
of the country of origin.

Every effort has been made to ensure that the information in the book is accurate.
The information in this book will be relevant to the majority of people but may not
be applicable in each individual case so it is advised that professional medical advice
is obtained for specific health matters. Neither the publisher nor author accept any
legal responsibility for any personal injury or other damage or loss arising from the
use of the information in this book. Anyone making a change in their diet should
consult their GP especially if pregnant, infirm, elderly or under 16.

www.orionbooks.co.uk

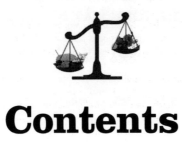

Contents

Thanks to ...

Araminta, Peta and Sophie for being there at the start of the 5:2 journey. Together, we're a lean, mean, slimming machine.

To all the fabulous members of the 5:2 Diet Facebook group, and especially to the people who told me everything about their diet history, health concerns and experiences of fasting. Thanks especially to Linda for her great graph and insights, and Jenny M for her fantastic response to the early draft.

To Fena Lee in Singapore for making the cover idea a reality.

To Amanda and the starry team at Orion for making this happen so fast.

To my parents for teaching me to love food and eating out.

To Rich for making me step away from my desk occasionally to eat, sleep and think about something other than fasting.

Special thanks to the BBC 'Horizon' team, and Dr Michael Mosley in particular, for making a programme that inspired so many people to try this approach to food and health.

Most of all, we all owe thanks to the many scientists who are pioneering so much incredible work in the field of fasting and health. We are hungry to see what you come up with next ...

What readers say about
The 5:2 Diet Book:

'Love this book! Having followed the 5:2 plan myself for a number of weeks, it was great to find this really helpful guide to use as support for when the going gets a bit tough! I really like the ease of following this diet plan, and it is working for me (10lbs weight loss in 8 weeks and counting, hopefully). This is an excellent tool to help you achieve your goals, whether they be weight loss, health or both. Thank you, Kate, for providing a friend to help me focus along the way!'

'Being a reasonably fit, sporty male, I was as interested in the long-term health benefits as the potential weight loss. Kate Harrison's book is written in an extremely readable style, the science is explained in a non-baffling way, and it's full of motivational tips and examples (as well as ideas for low-calorie menus/dishes that you don't need to be Jamie Oliver to prepare). Inspirational reading!'

'With Kate's help, I survived the fast days. I have heard so many success stories so keeping my fingers crossed but as it promises health benefits too, it can't be wrong! It is informative but humorous, it clearly states the facts but also shows that it is challenging but also very uplifting experience at the same time. It is good to read her experiences and the other people's. The recipes are good and I will definitely refer back to it ...'

'I'm a young(ish) man (32). I found this book very easy to read and am eager to start my own 5:2 diet. The resources are great with lots of ideas. For anyone who is new to this idea, this book is a great introduction.'

'It filled me with enthusiasm which doesn't happen often when I'm embarking on another diet. I'm now looking forward to getting into skinny jeans as I hit the 50 year old mark!'

'Fantastic book. Have tried this and it really works. If you buy one book in an attempt to lose weight this year make it this one. You will not regret it! I have tried everything over the last twenty years and this is the only way of dieting that I am able to stick with. The health benefits show pretty quickly too.'

'Well written book by someone who has been struggling with weight issues for most of adult life, like many of us. This makes it easy to relate, and easy to read. I will try the "diet" as soon as I'm back to work after holidays. New year, New body!'

'Kate's honest & easy to read guide helped me through the first fast day. When I felt wobbly I read the book! I loved the chatty way she takes you through and shares her journey. If you are contemplating the 5:2, this should be your bible.'

All reviews for the Kindle edition

Why reading this book will revolutionise your body and your future

Imagine a diet that lets you eat the foods you love,
most of the time.

That enables you to lose weight steadily.

That could reduce your risk of cancer, heart disease,
diabetes and Alzheimer's.

That makes your brain sharper and your
body more efficient.

That changes your attitude to hunger and food for ever.

A diet that involves no special 'low-cal' or 'lite' foods
and will save you money.

That's completely flexible, to fit your lifestyle.

That suits men and women, those new to diets
and those who've tried everything.

A diet you'll want to stick with for life.

Stop imagining. The 5:2 Diet is real.

January 2013

Dear Reader,

Six months ago, I watched a TV programme that changed my life.

I almost didn't write that line, because it sounds so cheesy, but it happens to be true. Sixty minutes of viewing set the scene for a huge change in my attitude to dieting, introduced me to an exciting new branch of medical science – and gave me the tools to begin transforming my body.

Of course, I've had to do the hard work myself, but the programme opened the door to the world of intermittent fasting and calorie restriction – the official name for an approach to health and diet which is gaining huge numbers of followers around the world. Many of them share their experiences for this book – experiences that are likely to inspire you to follow their lead!

What I've learned has made me feel in control of food, not the other way round. It's given me new hope that I can do something constructive to reduce my chances of developing cancer, dementia and diabetes, which have had devastating effects on members of my family. It's a lifestyle I want to follow … well, for life.

The rapid popularity of this approach is typical of many hyped diets. You know the ones. They're flavour of the month, and then they drop out of fashion almost as quickly.

But intermittent fasting is one diet craze that is anything BUT crazy

It's sustainable, adaptable and it might help you live longer. It's also very simple, and the 'fasting' part isn't nearly as punishing as it sounds because – whisper it – you never have to have to go a day without eating. You simply work one, two or more days of low-calorie eating into your weekly routine, and forget all about 'dieting' the rest of the time. Until you step on the scales or try on the jeans that didn't fit two weeks ago ...

And it's not just about how you look or how much you weigh – it's also about how your body works, right down to cellular level

Reducing your calorie intake radically for short periods, triggers changes in your body's metabolism and brain function that can cut the risk of the diseases we all fear: cancer, heart disease, Alzheimer's and diabetes. There are benefits for your body and your brain as your body works hard to repair cells damaged by lifestyle and ageing.

The 'diet' for people who don't diet

The health benefits are so great that people are choosing to adopt this approach to eating even if they don't have weight to lose – in my case, as I near my ideal weight, I have no intention of stopping. I'm going to carry on with the lifestyle because of the changes it's making. I have more energy than I have had in years, my outlook is more positive and I feel – and look – younger.

The approach helps you to change your attitude to food and eating for the better. In fact, many people prefer not to call it a diet at all, because so many calorie-controlled diets fail. It doesn't matter one bit whether you call this a diet/ way of eating/approach/lifestyle – what matters is that it's sustainable, sensible and intuitive. And it works.

The benefits of fasting have been known in medical circles for some time, but finally this way of eating is going mainstream

There are no hidden gimmicks, no complications, no over-priced supplements or revolting meal replacements. In fact, this way of eating will save you money.

Definitely not just for girls …

This is a diet that both men and women are adopting whole-heartedly, because it's so flexible and fuss-free. Fast Days offer a 'mini break' from worrying about food – and because you only have to be careful for a couple of days a week, you don't feel deprived. Plus, research suggests that even when you're given total freedom to eat what you like on Feast Days, dieters simply don't binge or over-compensate on the 'Feast' days. That's borne out by my own experience and that of hundreds of others I know who are doing this – we adopt healthier habits without even thinking about it.

The ultimate practical guide to the most sustainable diet there is.

The 5:2 Diet Book has all the information you need to start tomorrow. Or – if you're reading this before breakfast – you could even start today!

The book takes you step-by-step through embracing a lifestyle that suits your needs and goals. There is no proscriptive list of dos and don'ts, no list of 'Banned' or 'Sinful' foods. You work out the maximum number of calories you can eat on your Fast Days – then stick to that limit for a couple of days a week (or once a week, or every other day – it depends what suits you and how much weight, if any, you want to lose). Then you eat normally the rest of the time.

If it's that simple, why do I need a book about it?

Well, maybe you don't – if you stick to 500 calories a day (if you're a woman) or 600 (if you're a man) on your 'fast' days, then you'll almost certainly benefit.

But, when I started following this regime, I did have lots of questions and uncertainties and I looked in vain for a guide that would help me find the right approach.

Why I've written this book

Once I'd distilled all the information I could find, for my own use, I decided it would make sense to put it together and create the consumer guide I couldn't find... so here it is.

It'll be your companion when you start, with lots of practical information, recipes, meal plans and encouragement to help you launch this way of life and alter your body and approach to food for good. Pretty soon, this way of life should feel like second-nature – but the case studies and the remarkable scientific research underpinning this diet should help keep you on track. I've surveyed dozens of other 5:2 dieters, male and female, of all ages, who share their wisdom, successes and excitement about the changes they've seen.

I'm no doctor. I'm just a failed dieter who has found something that works for me, at last. And I am pretty certain it can work for you too. I happen to be a vegetarian and a 'Great British Bake Off' addict, but whether you're a dedicated foodie, or not fussed about cooking . . . a cuddly carnivore or a gluttonous veggie . . . a homebody or a party animal, you can make this fit your life.

Health warning

I have no medical training, though I've always taken a keen interest in food and nutrition. I'm going to share my experiences, and those of other successful 5:2 dieters.

But there are people who shouldn't follow this diet: children and teenagers; pregnant women; people with compromised immunity. If you have Type 2 diabetes or any other pre-existing conditions, you should talk to your doctor as this diet could help but you need to do it under supervision.

In addition, anyone with a history of eating disorders should definitely not undertake this without talking to their doctors.

In fact, even if you are otherwise healthy, talk to your GP – they're on your side, and if you are committed to losing weight, it'll make their job easier as your general health is likely to improve! It's also quite likely they'll know all about 5:2 – more and more doctors are so impressed by the science that they're trying it for themselves!

I have also included links for information and interest but please note, I am offering them for information only and I have no control over their content.

How this book works

The 5:2 Diet Book has three parts. **Part One** explains the thinking behind the diet – including medical and psychological research about why losing weight this way can boost your body in some incredible ways. These chapters alternate with my own diary, where I share highs and lows I encountered as I adapted to this new way of thinking about food and diet.

Part Two contains all the practical information you need to make 5:2, 4:3, 6:1 or Alternate Day Fasting (ADF) work for you. I've included information on how to prepare for the Fast Days and how to stay motivated, plus guidance on exercise and calorie counting, along with loads of real-life success stories and experiences to keep you on track.

Part Three focuses on food ideas for your Fast Days, with lots of simple options for meals and snacks to appeal to all tastes, including suggestions for seasonal eating and sample menus to stop you feeling hungry. I know preparing food when you're on a diet can be a chore, so there are also ideas from 5:2 fans who've suggested their favourite ready-made meals. Many of us prefer to leave cooking till 'Feast' days when you're free to make the dishes you love! But there are also satisfying recipes should you want to make all of your food from scratch.

At the end, I've included a **resources section** for further reading, including chapter by chapter links to articles that offer more detail on relevant topics. I've abbreviated the links to make them easier to type into your browser if you want to find out more by going online! Alternatively, you can download a single list of links free via the 5:2 website – *www.the5-2dietbook.com.*

And the last item of all is the final instalment of my diary, updated to include progress over the festive season and the New Year – keeping the weight off during family celebrations has proved far easier than I ever expected.

The simplest, most grown-up diet in the world

This diet – and this book – treats you like an adult. Pick and choose what makes sense to you. A lot of the science is new and evolving, so there are some questions which don't yet have definitive answers. My job is to offer you all the options so that, like me, you can find your own personalised way of working intermittent fasting into your life.

But have no doubt – this is working for thousands more of us. News of the diet is spreading far and wide – because it works. And it could work for you too.

Of course, I love feeling slimmer, but this is about much more than vanity. Like most of us, I know that there are many diseases like cancer and diabetes that have blighted my family – now at last I feel I can try something practical to improve my odds.

This book isn't about rules. It's about freedom. What's stopping you?

Kate Harrison

1

THE

5:2

REVOLUTION

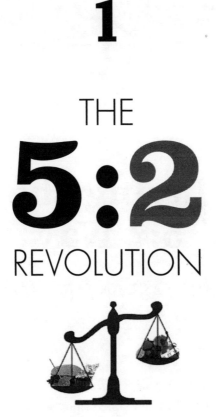

What the diet does, how it works, why it's for you

CHAPTER ONE

Living the 5:2 Way

FEAST, FAST AND BE HAPPY!

I am on a diet. But this one is different.

No, really. I understand your scepticism. I've spent almost two-thirds of my life on a diet. And 99% of my *adult* life either dieting or feeling rubbish about how I look.

I'm not unusual. Most women I know – and increasing numbers of men – have a love/hate relationship with their bodies and with food. OK, we can blame Size Zero film actresses for giving us unrealistic expectations about how we should look (and sending us to the biscuit tin for comfort). Or we could pin it on multi-national food companies or takeaway joints for trying to get us to eat more, more, MORE!

But short of avoiding Hollywood movies and growing all your food from scratch, there's little we can do about the external causes of what the press call the Obesity Epidemic.

What we *can* do is find a way of eating that works for us.

And – to my astonishment – I think I might have done that at last, at the ripe old age of forty-four.

For me – and many others you'll hear from in this book – it's *revolutionary.*

What life is like on 5:2

For breakfast this morning, I savoured a chocolate and almond croissant from the best bakery I know, the one that's tormented me with its forbidden treats since I moved into a house approximately thirty-five steps from its doors.

Except it doesn't torment me any more. Because thanks to the 5:2 Diet, I know I can indulge – even, occasionally, over-indulge – but still lose a significant amount of weight.

Tomorrow I'll be fasting, one of two Fast Days a week (the 2 in 5:2) when I make a big change. Strictly speaking, this isn't a true fast, because I can eat up to three small meals – but most 5:2 dieters do call these reduced calorie days Fast Days.

I will eat roughly 25% of the calories my body actually needs: at that level, the way my metabolism works will change, but I won't feel faint or unbearably hungry, as I might with a 'true' fast.

I'll most likely eat at lunchtime and dinner time: as it's winter, I'll probably have a soup for lunch, and a vegetable curry side dish for dinner, with some extra veg and perhaps a yogurt or a piece of fruit for pudding.

Yes, it *is* limited – but I don't care because the day after, I can forget counting calories and eat the things I enjoy.

Suddenly, food is all not about the Forbidden. I'm enjoying a balanced diet without feeling guilty about sharing a bottle of really delicious red wine, or having a full English for Sunday brunch.

So long as I keep a close eye on my eating habits for two days a week, I know I can enjoy a little of what I fancy the rest of the time – and still lose weight.

Since I discovered this way of eating just over five months ago I've lost over twenty pounds (9kg), without cutting out any of the foods I love: cheese, chocolate, the odd cocktail (make mine a Mojito). I haven't gone crazy – I probably have shifted to a more balanced diet on my five 'normal' days, but without making conscious changes. I simply have a much greater awareness of what my body needs, and when. I eat when I'm hungry and without bingeing.

And I savour every mouthful.

But food is only part of the picture. I wake up with much more energy, my mood is positive even though I'm writing on a wet and windy January day, and I feel relaxed but in control.

Don't just take my word for it...

I've surveyed dozens of dieters who are changing their lives for good.

When Linda first contacted me in November 2012, she'd just fasted for the first time, having tried numerous diets over the years. She was planning to fast twice a week, and joked that if it worked, she'd be running marathons at the age of one hundred.

Or at least, I thought she was joking. Now it's January and given her amazing progress so far, I think she's on track.

> *I've lost 2 stone 4 pounds. I'm now 10 stone so I wouldn't want to lose more than another 10 pounds. I've been doing 5:2 or 6:1 some weeks and I certainly aim on fasting one day a week for the rest of my life once I've lost the weight. I used to be really sluggish and generally had a nap in the afternoons (I'm 63 and retired) but now I've started the Couch to 5K running programme (I'm on week two) and I aim at walking two miles each day on the days I'm not running. I've started running or walking rather than catching buses.*
>
> LINDA, 63

This works for all ages and both sexes. Software architect Andrew and his five workmates all decided to begin the diet at the same time. Like many men, none had followed 'named' diets before, but were inspired by the simplicity and science of this approach. They've been tracking their progress for fourteen weeks now:

> *I have lost 5kg over 14 weeks, this seems to put me well within my target healthy weight. We have noticed how less tired we feel and how the diet has become easy to do. In fact we all look forward to our diet days. Overall we have lost about the same but the point of the 5:2 diet*

is not really about losing weight, it's about health. The
improvement in blood pressure, cholesterol etc. is why
we are doing it.

ANDREW, 42

Five kilograms is eleven pounds – an impressive loss. But how are they finding it? Thirty-four-year-old Sunil began the diet with a very clear target:

My main motivation is to reduce my cholesterol – I'm
a British Indian, so live mostly on an Indian diet
which isn't the best for reducing cholesterol. I wanted
to try a diet that doesn't have a major impact on my
life and this fits the bill. It's so easy. The first week or
two are not hard, but it just takes a little discipline. I
now don't even think about hunger on starving days.
It feels normal. I find that my general appetite is
less throughout the week – I used to have the urge to
binge in evenings after dinner. I've lost 3.2 kilograms
and added an extra notch to my belt. I'm getting my
cholesterol tested soon.

Forty-one-year-old software engineer Kostas has always been athletic, but has still struggled with blood pressure and weight concerns. Until now.

I've lost 2 kilos, feel much better (psychologically), less
bloated so I fit better in my clothes. The diet works,
and there are hundreds of meals you can plan during

a fasting day. The diet is keeping us healthier without depriving us of anything. Eventually, it will become a way of life. Now, even during my non-fasting days I am aware of what I eat and how much. I don't feel that I restrict myself from any kind of food that I like, because I can tell myself that I can eat it in my non-fasting days. My fasting days feel like I am cleansing myself.

The freedom – and the cost savings – appeal to Myfanwy, who has lost nine pounds. She was only slightly overweight to begin with and the loss has been steady. She's also showing a steady and welcome reduction in her blood pressure.

In terms of weight I am delighted to be slimmer and be able to wear things I never dreamed I would again. I can fit the diet around my life – work, teenage children, meals out, celebrations. It costs me nothing – and saves me money (no lunches or snacks on fasting days). There's no complicated calorie balancing and no inevitable guilt when one cannot keep a diet up day after miserable day.

MYFANWY, 49

The flexibility of the approach means people are trying out different variations – several of the men I've surveyed have gone for a stricter fast, for simplicity and speed:

I have had limited success with restricted calorie diets in the past, but was unable to keep up with them as a lifestyle. In under four weeks I've lost lots of weight and 2 inches off my waist. I love it! No calorie counting makes it much more sustainable for me. I believe it's much easier to water fast on fasting days than to consume the 500–600 cals that some do.

ROB, 42

The healthiest Diet?

So far, so good. We're losing weight and inches, and feeling motivated.

But there are other, even more important reasons why many of us have decided to do this diet:

My mother had every illness under the sun and I don't want to follow in her footsteps. I have a young family and wish to be around, plus weight loss and memory improvements would be a bonus. I've already lost two stone and inches from the stomach (which would suggest a reduction in the risk of heart disease). Plus, no saggy skin and my boobs have stayed the same size, even though they're usually the first to go on a diet!

FIONA, 41

I wanted to lower my blood pressure and cholesterol and after two months, so far, so good. It's easy and the more you do it, the easier it gets. I like that it makes scientific sense.

PAUL, 47

I'm doing this for weight loss and for health reasons. My father has Alzheimer's, plus I have high blood pressure.

SARAH, 49

Like Fiona and Sarah, I have concerns about my family's medical history, particularly diabetes and cancer. I'm still too young to be part of the official UK screening programme, but have mammograms every year because so many of my female relatives have developed cancer, including my mother, my aunt and my grandmother.

But what I've learned since I began to research this diet, has given me fresh hope. To give just one example: a major study has put women of my age, with the same increased risk of breast cancer, on a 5:2 style diet, with very encouraging results. The women have recorded good weight loss – which in itself helps to reduce the risk of developing various cancers. However, the researchers are also hoping that this kind of intermittent fasting might produce changes that work specifically to reduce the risk of breast cancer.

The study highlights additional improvements in how the women's bodies response to insulin – which also feels incredibly relevant to me as I am at very high risk of developing Type 2 diabetes, with all the complications that can involve.

Whatever medical conditions your family is prone to, there's an excellent chance that 5:2 eating may be beneficial. This approach hits the jackpot because of the incredibly powerful effects it has on your body – and your brain.

The Diet that succeeds where others have failed?

The diet works brilliantly for all adults, but anecdotally, it seems it's proving especially popular among those aged 35+. It is around this age that we often begin to find it tougher to shift excess weight. We also become more aware of our own mortality and of the health issues our parents or other family members are facing.

> *Couldn't fit in my clothes, saw my photos at my brother's 50th (awful), where we're all overweight, worried about joints etc, scared of being disabled through fatness. Mum is losing her short term memory and if fasting staves that off, I will give it a whirl. I need my brain. Feel a bit more hopeful of avoiding some of the health issues affecting my parents (and my grandparents before they passed away).*
>
> LINDA, 52

A Facebook group I set up (facebook.com/groups/the52diet – do pop in and say hello there or in our new forum at the 5-2dietbook.com) is full of motivating stories from men and women of all ages and occupations – and they're reporting the same great results. Not just weight loss, but also a feeling that you're doing something positive for your body.

Because the 5:2 diet has a huge advantage over other diets – it brings about physiological changes that help the body – and even the brain – heal itself.

Fasting does put stress on our systems but the way we

respond to that stress seems overwhelmingly positive. Research in humans and animals shows that fasting tends to lower the production of the IGF-1 hormone, which plays a role in the development of cancer. Intermittent fasting activates processes that repair the body's cells and cuts insulin production which in turn makes us less likely to lay down fat stores.

The effects on the brain are equally exciting. They include a potential reduction in the risk of Alzheimer's disease and other forms of dementia. On a more immediate basis, many people notice a lift in their mood, and fasting may even help with depression.

These long-term medical effects are, of course, harder to measure on an individual basis than weight loss – but increasingly evidence suggests this way of eating has positive effects that far exceed the benefits of weight reduction alone.

I've gone into the medical research and the science in Chapters Three and Four – it makes fascinating *and* motivating reading.

Back in control

There's another benefit that didn't feature in the BBC 'Horizon' TV programme, but has transformed the attitudes and lives of many 5:2 dieters.

This year, I'd more or less resigned myself to being fat and frumpy for ever. I felt out of control, and very depressed about my lack of willpower – yet I couldn't seem to find a way to overcome that.

To my surprise, my Fast Days have had a profound effect on

the way I think and behave, and not only when I'm consciously restricting calories. The experience of reconnecting with my appetite, and re-learning how to deal with occasional hunger pangs, has helped me and many other people get back in touch with how our bodies work.

> *I find fasting days very 'cleansing'. It has also made me realise that I can survive on a lot less calories than I thought I could. And periods of excess, e.g. Holidays, Christmas etc. can be 'put right' relatively effortlessly.*
>
> CLAIRE, 43

> *Working really well for me. I like the discipline on two days (and the self-awareness of slight hunger discomfort), combined with complete freedom the rest of the week.*
>
> JAMES, 43

I now believe very strongly that all those diets promising 'you'll never feel hungry' have done us a disservice. Knowing the difference between eating because you need to, and eating because you are bored/thirsty/fed up is a basic skill, and one that can help you control and understand your weight issues.

This way of eating has re-educated me about what my body needs, and when. Eating is less about habits and more about responding to my appetite: I'm not the only one to feel this way.

> *It's bloody easy, and it's good to feel hungry. From years of dieting lore that advocated eating little and often, it*

feels like a relief to be able to skip meals and breakfast particularly.

JULIA, 50

In Chapter Four I also delve deeper into the psychology of this lifestyle change.

The simplest Diet

The simplicity of this diet is what makes it so irresistible to many of us. You decide how many days a week to monitor calories – and then either do some basic maths to work out your 'limit' or simply opt for a goal based on average energy needs: 500 for women and 600 for men.

Then – you start. The foods you need on Fast Days can almost certainly be found in your cupboard, freezer, or definitely in your local supermarket. There's nothing specialised, no meal replacements or exotic supplements to be bought at huge expense.

I'm lazy when it comes to cooking so I keep things very simple – beans on toast for lunch and shop-bought soup for dinner. I won't be winning 'Masterchef' but I don't care because keeping it fuss-free is really important in staying on this diet.

KATY, 30

The only two tools that come in useful are a set of kitchen scales and either a calorie-counting book or access to the internet or a smartphone so you can use online tools or apps to calculate your intake. But even those aren't compulsory. If you follow the ready-made food suggestions in Part Three of this book, you'll be able to do the diet without extra calorie counting.

I tend to stick to Birds Eye chicken or beef dinners, or variations on that theme. They're all weighed out and have the calories on the boxes, so it saves weighing things and calculating calories.

SALLY, 49

I know pre-packed meals aren't for everyone, but it's much easier now to find dishes that are low in preservatives or other additives – and someone else has done the portion control for you.

The oldest Diet

Fasting is a part of almost all organised religions, suggesting that those faiths have long had an awareness of the benefits for mind *and* body of taking a break from eating, or alternatively eating very simply and frugally.

But you don't have to have any specific religious belief to follow the 5:2 diet – what you're doing is taking advantage of ancient wisdom that is now being validated by cutting edge research.

Not for everyone?

As I said in the introduction, there are groups of people who should not make such major changes in eating patterns including pregnant women or nursing mothers, children and teenagers, Type 2 diabetics, those with other medical conditions, and those who are either very lean or have a great deal of weight to lose. I do know some new mothers and morbidly obese people who are making this diet work, but it would be a very bad idea to begin without medical supervision.

The same applies to people with a history of eating disorders or psychological issues around food or appearance. For most of us, eating less on a couple of days a week is easy to adopt, but like any habit, it could be taken to extremes which could damage your mental or physical health. If you have any worries, please, *please* do talk to a specialist before considering the 5:2 or intermittent fasting approach.

Indeed, it's a good idea to talk to your GP about this, or any other dietary change. Sally is doing this already:

> *I'd suggest involving your doctor/practice nurse and going to be weighed there regularly too. That way they can keep an eye on you and a medical record of how the diet is affecting you. Most surgeries are set up to support weight loss.*

> SALLY, 49

I must admit I haven't gone down this route myself. I'd already been advised by my GP to lose weight and knew my basic health indicators – blood pressure, heart rate, fasting blood sugar – gave no particular cause for concern. But I did know I could count on their support to track the weight loss if need be. I'm looking forward to my next check-up so I can be told officially that I am in better shape! As you'll see in a moment, it's been a long journey …

In Chapter Two, I'll be talking about the maths of weight loss and how they relate to the 5:2 approach.

But before that, with apologies to Bridget Jones, here's the first of my 5:2 Diary entries, starting on the date that changed everything for me: August 6 2012.

Kate's 5:2 Diary Part One:

AUGUST 6 2012

A Couch Potato Watches TV & Makes a Decision

Weight 161 lbs/73 kg

Mood: guilty, resigned

Today I am the fattest I've ever been.

Even though I've started three diets this year alone, I keep getting bigger. I weigh eleven and a half stone (73 kg) – and am only five foot four inches tall (when I stand up *very* straight). So that gives me a BMI of 27.6 – and anything 25 or above is overweight. Eleven stone was bad enough – I thought that would be my mental limit, the moment where I took action, yet the weight is still creeping on.

My size 14 jeans (which I always tend to think of as a 16, as they're quite generously cut) are slicing into my waist, my bra is too tight and there are lumps and bumps showing when I wear anything but the baggiest of tops. Worst of all, my belly is wobbly – I've always been curvy, with big hips and boobs, but my tummy is now catching up.

Has anyone seen my willpower?

This is the slippery slope. I feel out of control, frumpy, middle-aged and very, very cross with myself. I don't want to be gaining half a stone a year, wearing a size 18 or more before

I'm fifty, feeling ashamed to go on the beach because I look like the fat lady on a seaside postcard.

Yet my willpower is diminishing with age, too. A few years ago, I managed to get to my lowest adult weight – a sylph-like eight and a half stone – thanks to low-carbing the vegetarian way. I felt good on it, wore skinny jeans for the first time, and really enjoyed eating lots of lovely cheese, Greek yogurt, nuts, berries and so on. And yet …

And yet even as people congratulated me on my success, a tiny part of me knew it couldn't last. I love bread, cakes and desserts. I have a huge recipe book collection and adore farmers' markets and nice restaurants, especially Indian or Italian places. Could I really turn my back on pasta, pilau rice and baked goodies for the rest of my life?

Plus, something didn't feel quite right about eating such a restricted diet: cutting out one food group seemed wrong.

Sure enough, the weight crept back on. I tried low-carbing again this last month, but I couldn't convince myself it was something that would last. Because, frankly, it won't.

Fat and fearful …

This is not simply about vanity anymore. Both my parents have Type 2 diabetes – the kind that is most often diagnosed in later life – and I've seen the complications it causes, especially to vision, joints and the circulation. Their diagnoses also mean my chances of getting it are very high.

Plus, there's the strong family history of breast cancer on Mum's side – and a friend who has recovered from breast cancer raised doubts about how reliant I was on dairy products on the low-carb veggie diet. Dairy is something she's minimised since she went into remission because she's concerned that too much of it might increase her cancer risk.

Though being overweight increases the risk of cancer, too. It's hard to know what to do for the best.

How much more desperate do I need to become?

I've joined a gym *again* and am trying to go, but, realistically, three cross-trainer sessions a week are going to burn 1,200 cals maximum. Apparently to lose a pound of fat, you have to cut 3,500 calories from your diet, or do 3,500-worth of activity without eating any extra food. Gym-going alone is not going to be enough. I've joined a website, MyFitnessPal.com, to monitor what I'm eating, but it's labour intensive and it doesn't include listings for the days I eat out, because it's impossible to know the calorie count of restaurant food.

Yesterday, I found myself Googling diet drugs – the kind that 'bind' to the fat you eat and help you pass it before it gets digested. The side-effects are utterly revolting and yet I went as far as filling in an online form to find out if I'd be eligible for them. I am, but apparently they're out of stock.

So I'm not alone in seeking a quick fix.

A Lost Cause …

Maybe I just have to accept this is the shape I'll stay. I could take down all the mirrors in the house to start with …

There's a BBC TV programme I'm going to watch tonight about fasting – the description of the show is intriguing. But let's face it – I don't have the willpower to do a 'normal' diet, never mind a fast. I suspect it'll just give me even more to feel guilty about.

10.05pm
Wow.

That was an amazing programme… really fascinating, full of counter-intuitive science and new information – plus fasting REALLY worked for the presenter.

Even better, it wasn't a 'true' fast – he did still eat on his fasting days, just an awful lot less.

The potential benefits also seem to go way beyond weight loss. There's a possibility that 'intermittent calorie restriction' – a more accurate but less catchy description than fasting – could reduce the risk of breast cancer, diabetes, heart disease and even Alzheimer's.

This is a diet that could offer more than weight loss alone.

But I have been here before, with low-carb, high-fibre, tum/bum/thigh. The fact is, miracle diets don't exist.

Or do they? Maybe this time, I might be able to get slim – and stay slim.

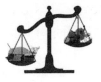

CHAPTER TWO

The Maths of Weight Loss – and why Fasting adds up

Slim people don't just look better by the pool.

They also live longer. The *rats*.

It's the reason your doctor monitors your weight and calculates your BMI – Body Mass Index – when you have a check-up. The BMI is a simple calculation based on your height and weight (some would say too simple: we'll talk about that a little later).

Broadly, if your BMI is over 25 – or 23 for some ethnic groups – you're officially overweight. And if it's over 30, you're classed as obese: the higher the figure, the higher the statistical risk of disease.

You can either calculate it by this formula, or by using the chart:

BMI = Weight (kg) / [Height (m) x Height (m)]

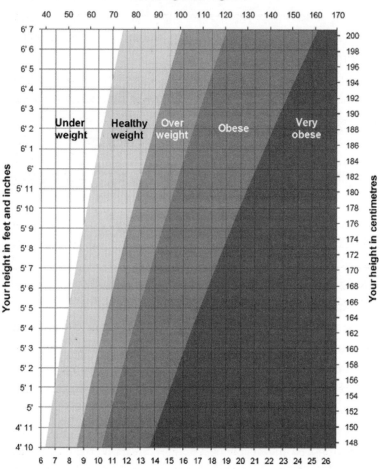

Your weight in kilograms

Your height in feet and inches

Your height in centimetres

Under weight

Healthy weight

Over weight

Obese

Very obese

Your weight in stones

BMI is far from perfect – you may have heard about rugby players or athletes who train for hours a day yet are classed as 'obese' by BMI standards because they have lean bodies with high muscle mass. BMI is also pretty hopeless in children. Plus, the risk calculations are based on large-scale studies so it can't tell you much about *your* personal specific risks, which depend on so many other factors: family history, genetics, lifestyle, environment.

Also, BMI isn't the only indicator of the effect excess weight could be having on your health. Your waist measurement is also a strong predictor of your likelihood of developing cardiovascular disease: it's an indicator of how much 'visceral' fat you've accumulated around the vital organs. This distribution of weight is important – 'pear' shaped people with larger hips and thighs tend to have lower risks than 'apples' who store more fat around the belly. The more you have, the higher your chances of developing heart problems or Type 2 diabetes. The current NHS guideline is that you are at greater risk if your waist (measured round your belly button) is more than 37 inches/94cm if you're a man and 31.5 inches/80cm if you're a woman.

Research presented at a conference in France in 2012 advises us to fine-tune that even more – by aiming to keep our waist measurements to less than half of our height. So, in my case, I am 64 inches tall, so my waist measurement should stay under 32 inches (it has fallen from 32 to 29.5 since I began the diet).

A six foot man (72 inches) should be aiming for a waist measurement under 36 inches. The research looked at data from 300,000 people and found the ratio between the two measurements was more effective at predicting the risk of diabetes, strokes and heart problems than the BMI – and if you measure your height in inches, it's very simple to do.

Lies, damned lies – and home truths?

Of course, the risks are calculated based on averages – and we all hope we'll be the exception to the rule. But before you write off the BMI or the waist circumference guidelines, remember statistics don't tend to lie. For every chain-smoking Great Aunt Winifred, who was the size of a horse and ate like one, and celebrated her 100th birthday with a bottle of gin for breakfast, there are millions of us whose diets are damaging our health.

Excess weight can increase our risk of developing a range of diseases and conditions including:

- High blood pressure
- Type 2 diabetes
- Coronary heart disease
- Strokes
- Gallbladder disease
- Cancer of the breast or colon
- Osteoarthritis
- Respiratory problems

Of course, you could hope you're going to be the exception that proves the rule. Or you can try to maintain to a 'healthy' weight to keep the statistics on your side.

Whatever your BMI, the truth is you probably don't need a figure to tell you you've put on too much weight. My guess is that if you're reading this book then you, like me, want to reduce your risks of these life-shortening, or quality-of-life reducing, conditions.

As well as looking better by the pool…

But, as we all know, losing weight is easier said than done:

I was first taken to a slimming club at the age of 11 and have been dieting ever since, sometimes with success, sometimes not. I originally lost weight when I was 17 by starving. I would have 1oz All Bran (dry) in the morning, an apple lunch time and plain salad in the evening. I used to tell my mum I was having lunch at college so that I didn't have to eat in the evening. I did this for 2 years and got down to 8 stone which is too thin for my 5 foot 7 inches! Once I started eating normally again the weight piled on. In my mid 20's I went to a slimming club and got to within 7lbs of my goal weight. Again, as soon as I started eating normally the weight piled on! Then Weight Watchers – Slimming World, Rosemary Conley classes, Atkins, Paul McKenna, Scarsdale … far too many diets to mention!!!

JEANNY, 53

I've tried all sorts – from The Cabbage Soup diet, Slimfast and the Beyoncé diet to Weight Watchers. The one that's worked best for long term weight loss was WW. I've had two successes there, though gradually the weight has gone back on. I'm greedy, really, it's that simple.

SARAH 49

Eating too much makes you fat – and other annoying things thin people say

People who don't struggle with their weight often have a maddening habit of stating the obvious.

'Losing weight is easy,' they'll say. 'Couldn't be simpler. Eat less, move more.'

Or they might point out the basic maths – that if you consume more food (or calories) than you burn off, you'll put weight on, and if you do the opposite then you'll lose it.

'Oh, if I feel a bit chubby,' they might say, pinching the imaginary inch (more like a millimetre) around their waists, 'I just hold off the chocolate for a couple of weeks and I'm back to normal.'

Well, bully for them! For many of us, it's a lot more complicated.

Don't blame yourself, blame biology

There are a whole range of reasons, a lot of them external. But one important internal factor is our biology: we are designed to take in as much energy as we can in the 'good' times, to help us survive in the leaner times.

It's only very recently that starvation has ceased to be a threat to most developed populations. Now, we have the widest choice of foods available to us – including all the healthy, fresh, minimally processed foods that doctors and diet experts recommend.

So why do so many of us make such bad choices?

Because our bodies still act as though we're living in caves, rather than centrally heated houses, and still work as though we have to hunt and gather our food, instead of nipping to the supermarket or even ordering our groceries online. What that means is, we naturally crave high energy foods.

Our bodies can't think ahead. All they can do is react to now. So when sweet and fatty foods are on offer, we're programmed to like the taste and texture, and to eat as much as possible – so we can lay down fat stores for a nutritional 'rainy day'.

For our ancestors that made perfect sense, because there were plenty of times when there was no food to be had, so we relied on the times when we'd eaten everything that was available, to store energy for survival.

But now, even if the economy is suffering, we tend not to cut back on food. And we still crave the sweet, fatty stuff.

Some people do manage to strike a balance, and stay slim. However, increasing numbers of us are becoming overweight or obese. And we need a new strategy to help cope with external factors like those glamorous air-brushed actresses, enticing new foods and energetic marketing.

Turning biology to your advantage

What 5:2 and fasting does is to go back to basics – I think of it as reintroducing some of the 'rainy days' our ancestors were only too familiar with, by providing less energy from food, in a controlled way.

How the body responds is incredible, as we'll see in Chapter Three. More and more experts are convinced it's what we were designed to do. But the mind adjusts well, too. Fast Days are limited, but Feast Days allow us to enjoy food, including the dishes we love, without feeling guilty. You might expect to binge, but research shows you rarely do. And if you shed the guilt, you begin to eat like a slim person. Here's what Sally has to say about it:

> *I like the idea that no foods are sins. As a lifetime yo-yo dieter, I've found something that really works for me. It isn't too hard to fit it into my lifestyle as it's flexible, and if I can't fast one day for any particular reason (i.e. a social occasion) I don't feel that I've failed. I just start again the next day.*
>
> SALLY, 49

I'm the same: within a couple of weeks I no longer felt deprived, or guilty, or ruled by my emotional response to food. As I felt less guilty, I was much more in touch with eating what I needed and no more.

Which meant weight loss became less about the psychology and more about the maths.

5:2: just a different way of eating less?

On the simplest level, 5:2 – or 6:1 or 4:3 or ADF – appears to work the same way as every other diet – you lose weight because you consume less energy (food) than you're using. The weight loss comes because, overall, you're eating less.

It doesn't sound very exciting – though some of the other physical and mental effects really are – but, ultimately, it's the same with all diets. It is possible that with fasting – as well as some other diets – there's what's known as a *metabolic advantage:* that is, eating this particular way will generate more weight loss (or, more specifically, *fat* loss) than can be attributed to the reduction in calories. But further research is needed.

Until we have more data, calories count on all diets. Take low-carbing. There's lots of talk about ketosis, which is a state where the body begins to access stored fat for energy because it's run out of the easier-to-process sugars it usually has access to when we're eating carbohydrates. Those behind various low-carb regimes say that ketosis is one of the key factors in the weight losses observed by followers: it is seen by some almost as a 'magic' state.

However, many studies have shown that it's much more straightforward than that. Low-carb dieters are consuming fewer calories than they did before, simply because they've cut an entire food group out of their diet.

That's what happened to me when I did low-carb. I ate less, without really thinking about it, because I had fewer choices. Yes, I could eat butter, which I love, but what was the point without crusty bread or a lovely hot baked potato? I didn't feel hungry, particularly, because protein tends to make you feel fuller, which is one advantage of a high-protein diet (there are potential disadvantages, too, as we'll see elsewhere). Of course, low-carb diets are also often high in fat, which is another factor: all that fat made me feel a bit sick after a while and I didn't want to eat anything at all. Therefore, I was eating less calories, almost by default.

But as soon as I started reintroducing the breads and potatoes into my diet (we moved to Barcelona, where 'pan con tomate' is served everywhere, and potato-packed tortilla is the default vegetarian option), I was no more able to resist them than I was before.

I boomeranged right back to my previous weight. And then some. Among the slim young things of one of Europe's funkiest city, I felt like a terrible frump. Which made me eat more.

The more extreme diets – Cabbage Soup, Maple Syrup, Grapefruit – cut your calorie intake by restricting your diet, but also your social life. Would anybody want to live on grapefruits for the rest of their life? I think it would feel like a very, very long life.

And as for cabbage soup … let's not go there.

But the bottom line about most diets is that they take the pleasure out of food.

The basic dieting equation:

X (the energy your body needs to function) minus Y (3,500 calories)
= Z (a weight loss of 1lb or 0.45kg)

As you can tell, algebra has never been my strong point. But simple arithmetic I *can* do.

And it works like this. It's estimated that to lose a pound of weight, we need to have a 'deficit' of 3,500 calories – the same figure applies to putting weight *on*. If we eat 3,500 more calories than we need – over any period of time – we will potentially weigh a pound (0.45 kg) more. That helps to explain why even eating one extra biscuit a day, for example, can lead to significant weight gain over a year. On the positive side, it also means small cuts in our daily consumption – not taking sugar in hot drinks, say – can have impressive cumulative effects.

So, to become a pound (0.45 kg) lighter, you must eat 3,500 less calories than your body needs (throughout this book, when I refer to calories, I'm referring to what nutrition labels list as kilo calories or kcal.). Eat 35,000 calories fewer and that's ten pounds (4.5 kg) gone.

That's the theory. As with everything in the diet/nutrition world, not it's not quite that simple. A calorie is a simple measure of energy, but it doesn't reflect the different ways the body processes calories from fat, carbohydrate and protein, which can affect how we store excess calories.

Another factor in how much weight we might lose is exercise – we're encouraged to exercise as part of a healthy living plan, but muscle mass is denser and heavier than fat.

For the sake of simplicity, let's work with the 3,500 as it gives us a baseline. Whatever the exact numbers, it's very clear that to lose weight we must create a deficit to make our bodies turn to our fat stores for energy. The question is, how do you achieve this deficit?

For my entire dieting life, I've assumed that you must diet *all the time:* and that's where it's become tricky, because it's so hard to deny ourselves the foods we're programmed to crave. It's even harder to keep to a regime when all you can see ahead is more deprivation.

All that time, there has been another way

5:2 – and all other types of intermittent fasting/calorie restriction – offer a radically different, though surprisingly obvious, solution. If you reduce your calorie intake more drastically, but for a limited period, you'll lose the weight. Because you aren't denying yourself the pleasures of food – or the social aspects of eating – the whole time, you stand a much higher chance of staying on track. Plus, knowing the medical benefits motivates you still further. It's win-win.

> *My other half is a chef, and having smaller portions or calorie counting 7 days a week just ain't going to happen, but I can manage 2. To my mind the big benefit is the 5:2 is far easier to fit round family life/ socialising etc. as one doesn't have to worry about it for the vast proportion of the time.*
>
> SARAH, 49

Doing the math(s)

So let's look at it in purely numerical terms.

A moderately active, average-sized woman needs 1800–2000 calories per day to maintain her weight, while for men it's 2300–2500. This is known as the Daily Calorie Requirement (there are instructions for calculating your own DCR in Part Two).

Let's use Miss Average as an example for now.

2000 (DCR) x 7 (days of the week) = 14,000 (total calorie needs to maintain current weight)

Conventional calorie-controlled diet

If you're overweight and want to lose a pound a week (which many doctors suggest as a 'sustainable' weight loss), you'd have to lower your intake by 3,500 calories i.e. consume a maximum of **10,500 in one week – which is 1,500 calories per day.**

This is how you'd aim to achieve that on a traditional calorie-controlled diet, where you're eating the same every day.

7 days at 1,500 calories per day

Weekly Total = 10,500 calories

That's actually a higher allowance than many calorie-controlled diets, but it still means calorie counting every day for a very long period: with a stone (14 lbs or 6.4 kg) to lose, for example, you're talking about fourteen weeks of counting and deprivation. If you're looking to lose four stone (25 kg), you're facing over a year of constantly obsessing over what you're eating. That's boring, anti-social and a constant reminder that you're 'different'.

5:2 Diet

Let's compare it to 5:2: you're cutting the calories more drastically for just two days of the week (or three or one, depending on what suits you best). The rest of the time you eat normally.

5 x Feast Days (approx. 2000 calories) = 10,000 calories

2 x Fast Days (500 calories = 25% of DCR) = 1000 calories

Weekly total: 11,000

In this example, you're eating 500 cals more than you would by calorie counting every day. This would potentially slow down weight loss slightly, though many dieters I've spoken to say that on Feast Days, they tend to naturally eat a little less – so I suspect it evens out.

But there's another crucial point about 5:2 – you don't actually need to calorie count the rest of the time. You can eat what you feel like.

Many people really can't believe this at first, but research has shown that ICR (intermittent calorie restriction) doesn't lead to bingeing. On average, ICR dieters eat between 95% and 125% of what they need – but even the higher figure isn't enough to cancel out the fast days.

I can fast because I know next day I can have chocolate AND wine if I so wish. Funnily enough, because I can, I don't binge.

MYFANWY, 49

My 'problem' is that having eaten low calorie foods for most of my life it's hard to eat anything like 'normal' calories on my 'feasting' days, so will often eat a couple of biscuits or have a glass of wine to make up the calories!

LINDA, 63

Of course, if you decide to do the diet more often than two days a week – every other day, for example (known as Alternate Daily Fasting or ADF) – the calorie deficit increases. So fasting on Sunday, Tuesday and Thursday looks like this:

4 x Feast Days (approx. 2,000 calories) = 8,000 calories
3 x Fast Days (25% of daily energy needs) = 1500 calories
Weekly Total: 9,500 calories

Many people on ADF do stick to three Fast Days – but it's advisable that you don't fast more often than every other day. There's a risk you'll get fed up with restricting so often – what you're looking for is a sustainable lifestyle.

What are the Fast Days like?

I won't lie – they can take some getting used to at first. We're so used to eating before we get anywhere near experiencing hunger that it can be odd or even alarming to begin with when our appetite kicks in.

> *It's easy, and the more you do it, the easier it gets. Eat some protein on your restricted days, give the regime at least a month before considering if it works for you or not.*
>
> PAUL, 47

> *I like the discipline on two days (and the self-awareness of slight hunger discomfort), combined with complete freedom the rest of the week. I've learned to enjoy the empty stomach feeling.*
>
> JAMES, 43

500 calories for women – and 600 for men – is enough to keep you from feeling unwell, especially if you choose your foods

wisely: there's much more about what to eat in Part Three.

Plus, believe it or not, hunger isn't a huge deal. When was the last time you felt hungry, instead of thirsty or bored? Allowing yourself to experience hunger – and to see how little food it takes to feel full again – is a huge help when you want to have more control over your appetite and your eating.

Finally, and crucially, *it's only one day at a time*. In contrast to the daily monotony of 'normal' diets, with 5:2 you're only having to limit yourself for a couple of days (and they're not consecutive). It's so much easier to say no to a cake or a glass of wine when you know you can have it tomorrow than it is when your diet feels like a very long punishment for being fat.

Weight loss is only the start ...

So the maths makes sense, and most people find this diet far easier to stick to than conventional calorie-controlled regimes (see the links list for research backing this up).

But 5:2 is about so much more than weight loss. The evidence that fasting brings physiological and mental changes is growing all the time. As we'll see in the 'science bit' in Chapter Three, the secret's in your cells and your genes.

But before that, find out how I got on in the first week of *my* fasting experiment ...

Kate's 5:2 Diary Part Two:

AUGUST 9 2012

First Fast – of many?

Mood: excited, apprehensive, unsure

I'm taking the plunge. Fasting is the future … maybe.

My boyfriend is sceptical, and other friends (who haven't seen the programme) are also dubious – one talked in dark tones about 'starvation mode' where your body responds to cutting calories by slowing down all its systems to keep you alive: that could mean when you go back to eating normal amounts, you put even more weight on.

But from my research online, the jury's out about whether that mode even exists. And if it does, then fasting one day at a time means you're not at risk of a metabolic 'go slow.'

If in doubt, *Google* it …

As I am self-employed, and work from home, my first response to pretty much all my daily decisions is to Google them. Seriously. It's not something I'm proud of – recently I've asked the big G where to rent a holiday cottage, how to answer my brand new but complicated mobile phone, and whether it's true that Marilyn Monroe was severely flatulent (apparently so). So it's inevitable that I'm doing the same with 5:2.

The TV show was fascinating, but I still have lots of questions: how many meals a day should I eat on the 'fast' days – is it better to eat one or three? What should my calorie target be on those days? Can I *really* eat as much as I like on my unrestricted or 'feed days'? Apart from eating slightly less, is the diet different for women?

I fully expected to find lots of sites dealing with this approach, but what's out there doesn't seem to be aimed at the layperson – I found either scientific papers or pretty intense body-building sites.

What I did read seems to back up the potential health benefits, though. Plus, having worked as a producer at the BBC myself, I know how stringent the guidelines are for making any health claim on a programme, so I am certain the ideas 'Horizon' featured will be sound – so I'm giving it a whirl.

Doing the Math(s)

The first thing I have to do is work out roughly how many calories I need to maintain my current (over)weight.

I could use the average fast day limit of 500 calories. But I'm keen to know exactly where I stand, so I use the calculators on the MyFitnessPal website. It's a very neat site which, so far, has mainly helped me record exactly how much I'm eating – too much – and made me feel guilty about my weekly intake of cava (what I really need is an app that stops me opening the bottle in the first place).

My first step is to work out my Basal Metabolic Rate – an estimate of how many calories I need just to get through the day. The calculator tells me it's 1,365 which is a terrifyingly low figure …

Then I realise that's based on just keeping all your body's systems ticking over. So I must factor in my activity level using the Harris Benedict Formula – which sounds a bit like an episode of *Sherlock*. Because I do some light exercise, I multiply my BMR by 1.375 which gives me … a more generous **1876.87.**

That's my daily calorie requirement (DCR) – the calories I should eat to stay at roughly my current weight. Except of course I've been putting it on. Goodness knows how many calories I've put away to be this big.

The third calculation is the most important – for my new regime to actually count as a fast (and potentially bring me all the health benefits that scientists are researching) I divide my DCR by 4.

It comes to a slightly scary 469.25 – even lower than the averages of 500 for women and 600 for men that presenter Dr Michael Mosley quoted on the programme. **(There's a full guide to calculating your DCR in Part Two.)** I go to the fridge and start reading labels – on ready meals, soups, fruit and veg packaging.

Yes, it's low. But it's also … possibly … doable.

Little and How Often?

My final decision is how often I'm going to calorie restrict. On Twitter, Dr Mosley said he's cut down from 5:2 to 6:1 because he was losing so much weight. Or for fast weight loss, there's alternate day fasting, but I'm a bit daunted by that. Right now,

I don't know how I'll cope with even a single day of eating less than 500 calories in total.

5:2 sounds like a good start. Now all I need to do is, well, start …

FAST DAY 1: AUGUST 9 2012

I wake up and try to pretend it's a normal day. A normal day where I happen to limit myself to a quarter of what my body needs, energy wise, and probably about a sixth of what it normally gets!

I eat the same breakfast most days – a mix of Greek yogurt and raspberries that I got to like when I low-carbed. It keeps me from feeling hungry till lunchtime. Trouble is, my usual portion size would take up more than half my calorie requirement for the day. So with the help of my digital scales, I measure out a doll-sized breakfast. If you've never tried measuring out 25g of yogurt, it's a *tiny* quantity, approximately one fifth of a small pot. Not very much. I use a tiny bowl and savour all four tea spoonfuls.

I've bought a big bottle of sparkling water, as my main 'treat'– also, I know as a diet veteran that staying hydrated is super-important. Looks like these are the only bubbles I'll be getting today …

As lunchtime approaches, my mood is not best helped by a rejection letter from the Women's Institute where I'd auditioned to be one of the speakers on their official list. I'd given talks to them in the past, but at my audition, the 100-strong panel decided I wasn't up to it – though they do say I had a clear speaking voice and a pleasant personality.

Hmm. Good job they can't see my grumpy face now, as I stand in the kitchen with the letter in one hand, the other one hovering over the packet of HobNobs.

But no.

I am better than that! And *pleasant,* too.

I make myself a calorie-free black coffee and try not to think about lunch. Or to swear under my breath in my clear speaking voice.

The Department of Weights and Measures

Weighing is good displacement activity. That, and reading the labels on the back of ready meals because I just didn't fancy cooking with so few calories to play with. I found a Butternut Squash dish in Marks & Spencer with just 140 calories for half a pack. OK, I think it's meant as a side dish, but it's quite filling for lunch and also allows me to treat myself to five cherry tomatoes, some rocket leaves and a teaspoon full of balsamic vinegar as a dressing.

And, to keep it simpler, I have the same for dinner. Why mess with a winning formula? Dessert is the same as breakfast. And the total: 463 calories! Three under, should have had a couple more rocket leaves…

Time for bed

How's it been? Well, I've got a slight headache but no other symptoms. In truth, I've felt more peckish than truly hungry. Portions are small but it's been easy because the man of the house is out with mates tonight, so I haven't had to cook or resist sharing some wine.

But mainly it's been easy because I know I can eat exactly what I want tomorrow. I go to bed early – my tummy is rumbling, but my conscience is clear, and I hope to dream of what I can eat for breakfast in just over 12 hours' time.

What I ate to the last gram:

Breakfast

Greek-Style Natural Yogurt,	25 g	34 cals
Ground Almonds	4 g	25 cals
Strawberries – Raw	53 g	17 cals

Lunch

M & S Moroccan Butternut Wedges		
With Roast Vegetables	½ pack	140 cals
Peppery Baby leaf Rocket Salad	20 g	4 cals
Balsamic Vinegar of Modena	5 ml	5 cals
Cherry Tomatoes	5 tomatoes	15 cals

Dinner

M & S Moroccan Butternut Wedges		
With Roast Vegetables	½ pack	140 cals
Cherry Tomatoes	5 tomatoes	12 cals
Generic – Balsamic Vinegar	0.25 tbsp	3 cals

Snacks

Greek-Style Natural Yogurt	19 g	25 cals
Ground Almonds	5 g	31 cals
Strawberries – Raw	63 g	12 cals

Total for day: 463 cals

CHAPTER THREE

The Fasting Recharge – make your body work better, and last longer

Weight loss is only part of the attraction of 5:2. This is the first 'diet' that appeals to people who aren't overweight but want to take advantage of the incredible health benefits that fasting offers.

Increasing numbers of studies on both humans *and* animals suggest that there are unique benefits to be gained from fasting or restricting your calorie intake quite severely, *even if you only do it some of the time.*

We are talking about short-term changes – more energy, lower blood pressure and harmful cholesterol readings, higher levels of concentration – as well as long-term effects that help prevent the diseases that can affect our lives profoundly.

No wonder the weight loss begins to seem like the least important benefit!

I have concerns over dementia as it runs in my family so this side was particularly appealing.

KIRSTY, 38

I've always eaten carefully in terms of nutrition but I am doing this for its possible health benefits. Alzheimer's, cancer, heart disease, high cholesterol, are all threats at my age. My cholesterol was 7.6, I have had breast cancer, my mother, at 94, has very poor memory.

ROS, 69

Why does this work?

Common sense might suggest that depriving the body of nutrients would be damaging and, indeed, it does put the body under stress.

But it's the body's response to that stress that seems to hold the key to the health benefits – just as a stressful job can bring out the best in us and help us achieve more, or we push ourselves in the gym and end up feeling better for it, putting your body under stress in a controlled way, can encourage it to heal itself and trigger processes that protect and repair.

Time for the science bit: the secret is in the cells ...

The science bit is short, and sweet, and if you want to understand why this diet might have such huge benefits, it's worth focusing on this part! I've found it very inspiring to discover what's going on when I fast.

But if you're not in the mood for theory, do feel free to leave reading this till later. Part Two is the practical part, and I want you to use, and abuse, the guide as it suits you. No rules, remember?

Still with me? Great. We're all made up of cells – approximately 100 million *million* of them in total. Think of TV images of 'test tube babies' and IVF where you can see the cells doubling in number over and over again, as the embryo develops.

Our cells continue their hard work throughout our lives. There are approximately two hundred different kinds, all with different functions – and they're being replaced at the rate of millions per second. Some cells are constantly replaced, though others can't be replaced. Even those that do multiply can only do so a certain number of times. It's this ceiling that is responsible for ageing – as the number of skin cells drops, for example, your skin becomes thinner.

As part of their life cycle, some cells will also self-destruct, in a carefully controlled house-keeping process known as **apoptosis** – they'll even 'tidy up' after themselves as they prepare to die so they don't leave behind anything that could damage other cells. I love the idea of cells doing a Girl Guide-style good turn for the body, even as they approach the bitter end ...

Another important process is **autophagy** – literally 'self-eating': this process can lead to the death of a cell but may also help it to survive under stress by recycling amino acids and removing damaged parts of the cell. The two processes work together to keep the body running efficiently.

But sometimes the cell production and destruction process goes wrong: when too many cells are produced, uncontrollably, it causes tumours. The kind that then invade neighbouring tissues are malignant – in other words, cancerous.

Meanwhile, damage to brain cells can cause Alzheimer's or other forms of dementia, as the structure of brain cells is changed: the cells may die or the pathways become tangled up, and the chemical messengers that pass information around the brain no longer work as efficiently.

The more I've read about the science, the more amazed I've become at how hard the body works to regulate and protect itself. But time still catches up with us in the end …

Living causes ageing

The trouble with life is that the very process of living causes damage to the body.

Cells are damaged by the processes involved in producing the energy we need to function – our bodies break down food into glucose (the simplest form of sugar) to use as energy, but that breaking down also damages proteins in the body and causes many of the signs and symptoms of old age.

Oxygen is a vital part of that process, of course, but while the body makes the energy, it's also producing free radicals which attack your cells in a process known as oxidative stress. When we're younger, we can cope better with this, 'mopping up' the free radicals before they do too much damage. But it catches up with us sooner or later …

Can eating less slow this down?

At the simplest level, if you produce less energy, then you're potentially also causing less damage. That's one of the fundamental issues at the heart of much anti-ageing research.

It's been demonstrated in animal studies – from fruit flies to worms, mice to dogs – that eating less, or less frequently, can prolong their lives.

The exact chemical and biological interactions involved are being researched, but the studies have already led to many people choosing to eat less than their calorie requirements, all the time – not just to keep their weight down, but to increase their lifespans.

As someone with a keen interest in diets and nutrition, I've read a lot about Calorie Restrictors – these people typically eat only 70–80% of their recommended intake, though they take extra care to eat very nutritious foods. Many people end up with BMIs of 19, 18 or lower, and frequently show reduced blood pressure and cholesterol levels. One of the main movements is called Calorie Restriction with Optimum Nutrition – which is why they're known as CRONIES.

However, what I had read and viewed on TV about CRONIES had put me off – the guy featured in the BBC 'Horizon' programme seemed fairly typical in that his diet looked expensive and pretty wasteful – he kept the skin of fruit for example but discarded the pulp. And though he was very healthy, living that way all the time didn't look much fun!

Now it seems 5:2 and Alternate Day Calorie Restriction may offer the benefits of that CRONIE lifestyle – but in a much more civilised and laid back form. Instead of having to watch calories obsessively all the time, we can do it in short, sharp bursts that encourage the body to activate all the protective and reparative processes that may help us live longer and better.

It's not just how much you eat, it's also what you eat

Different foodstuffs also have different effects on the body – we've already mentioned that producing glucose stimulates those damaging free radicals.

According to the 'Horizon' show, protein in particular seems to turbo-charge the cell production process. The scientist interviewed, Professor Valter Longo, compared our bodies to racing cars where protein is making the cars race faster – what Dr Mosley called Go-Go Mode – with no chance at all to retune or recharge. Driving at high speed the whole time without ever putting the cars in for service causes wear and tear – and so if we eat constantly, we're effectively increasing the wear and tear on our bodies.

So what fasting or severely limiting energy consumed from food does is put our bodies in for a service. We deprive our body of calories – fuel – and that way, instead of making the body produce new cells, we encourage it to take stock – and take care of – the cells it already has.

IGF-1 – the 1 to watch?

IGF-1 is a growth hormone that many scientists in this field believe is central to the effects of this diet, *and* to both the ageing process and the development of cancers. IGF-1 stands for Insulin-Like Growth Factor and it plays an important role in children's growth.

But once we're adults, the effects are not as positive: in particular, the hormone seems to lock us into this constant cycle of regrowth that may not do us any favours, the *go-go* mode Dr Mosley talked about.

There's firm evidence in animal studies that lower levels of IGF-1 can lead to better health and longer life expectancy: mice on a diet of either continuous calorie restriction or intermittent calorie restriction have been shown to live 40% longer than mice fed a normal diet: that would be the equivalent of a person living to 120 or more!

Indeed, a recent report also suggests that a hormone that blocks the action of IGF-1 might in future offer some of the longevity benefits of fasting or calorie restriction – without having to fast! A group of mice were genetically engineered to produce constant supplies of a hormone usually produced during fasting, FGF21. The experiment extended their lifespan by a third, although fertility and bone density were affected (for more detail about all these studies, refer to the links section at the back of the book).

The curious case of the people 'immune' to cancer

Of course, we need to be wary of assuming that what works in mice will work in the same way for us. One clue comes from a rare *human* genetic condition known as Laron syndrome, where very low levels of IGF-1 are produced. People with the mutation don't grow very tall, but the lack of the hormone also has very strong protective effects against cancer and diabetes. Professor Longo from the University of Southern California – the same guy who gave us the car analogy above – monitored 99 people with the condition in Ecuador with astonishing results.

To date, they've now been followed for twenty-four years, and none of them has developed diabetes, and only one has been diagnosed with non-fatal cancer. Yet 5% of their neighbours – with similar diets and lifestyles – have been diagnosed with diabetes, and 17% had cancer diagnosed during that same period. Overall, the Laron syndrome group didn't live longer, but that may be down to the high number of accidents caused by being smaller.

One pointer towards the possible protective effects of low-levels of IGF-1 came when the scientists studied blood serum from those with the Laron mutation under the microscope. Cells suffered less DNA damage than 'normal' blood cells from non-Laron patients when they were exposed to a toxin. Yet when the scientists added IGF-1 – that protection disappeared.

Food and IGF-1

So if IGF-1 is a contributor to DNA damage – the kind we talked about when we were discussing Free Radicals and Oxidative stress – then what happens when we eat less and consequently produce less IGF-1?

It seems that as levels of the hormone drop, the body goes into the repair mode we mentioned before. This amazing process is one we can trace right back to the way our ancestors lived.

Their lives involved the most extreme version of 'fasting' and 'feasting' – Tina put it so clearly when she wrote to update her progress since she's been doing 5:2.

> *If you think about it, it's the most natural way to eat and probably how our cavemen ancestors would have survived. They'd have hunted an animal, eaten their kill, and may not have caught another for a few days so would have eaten much fewer calories until their next catch.*
>
> TINA, 49

Our bodies adapted to those dramatic variations in food intake very efficiently – but as I said in my introduction, it means they are focused on laying down fat stores, which works less well for us in times of permanent plenty. So this way of eating simulates the same lifestyle – and scientists have focused on the actions of one particular gene that is key to the repair processes.

The SIRT1 gene – gene genius of anti-ageing?

That gene is called the SIRT1 gene and produces a protein, Sirtuin (*silent mating type information regulation 2 homolog*: don't worry, there won't be a test at the end). Calorie restriction and fasting seems to activate the gene, with life-extending and anti-ageing effects.

It certainly does the trick for yeast and worms. Having extra copies of this gene extends their lifespans.

In human-focused research, there's been attention paid to the effect of calorie restriction in activating the gene, and all the 'repair mode' benefits we've been discussing in this chapter.

The theory goes that Sirtuin may play a part in regulating/improving the processes we've discussed above, including apoptosis (regulated cell death), reducing damage by 'free radicals' and also reducing what's known as inflammatory response. That's where the body tries to protect itself from infection – it works well when you have a cut or a minor infection, and various infection-fighting cells cause inflammation including redness and swelling as they race to the location to fight the infection. But it's not good news when your body overall stays in this inflamed state – in fact, it's thought chronic inflammation might be responsible for many medical conditions, including cancers, heart disease and arthritis.

So a reduction in inflammation triggered by SIRT1 may be responsible for many of the benefits seen in animals and humans – and it can be activated by calorie restriction, including 5:2 and ADF diets. Further research is ongoing into this – and into the possibility that you can also give your SIRT1 gene a boot up the backside with ... red wine?

The wine connection

The skin and pips of grapes contain a molecule called resveratrol – and some scientists believe this might partly explain the 'French Paradox', where studies have shown French citizens live longer than other Western Europeans, despite diets high in fat.

But before you crack open the vin rouge, I have to tell you that the research is not conclusive and is ongoing – billions of dollars are being spent trying to use this knowledge to develop life-extending treatments. Yet the role of the resveratrol – and the SIRT1 gene in general – in increasing lifespans is still controversial.

Uncertainties and motivation

The precise mechanisms of SIRT1, resveratrol and IGF-1 in the fasting process are still unclear, but there are numerous studies showing the potential beneficial effects of ADF and calorie restriction on different medical conditions.

Research in this area is ongoing, but for me (and for most of the scientists involved), there's enough evidence from different sources to convince that the 5:2 (or 4:2, 6:1 or ADF) life is the way forward.

In the next section, I'll summarise some of the most exciting medical research – I've found this very motivating to flick through if the hunger pangs strike! Remember there are links to all the research in the section at the back, so you can follow up the areas that are of most interest to you.

Medical research on specific conditions

Much of the evidence at this stage comes from animal studies, because human lifespans are so much longer and therefore the studies take longer too. So where humans have tried ADF or Calorie Restricted Diets, the effects are often measured by blood tests that show chemical 'markers'. These indicate the likelihood of developing certain diseases, e.g. insulin sensitivity for diabetes and LDL and HDL cholesterol for heart disease.

The more this area of research grows, the more long-term information about the real-time results in human subjects should be available.

For an excellent overview of some of the best research in the field, Dr Krista Varady – who featured in the 'Horizon' programme – and Dr Marc Hellerstein put together a review of studies in 2007 – there's a link in the resources section.

Cancer

In animal trials, there are signs that ADF (and intermittent calorie restriction) has inhibited the growth of certain cancer cells, and improved response to anti-cancer therapy.

Meanwhile the Genesis Breast Cancer Prevention Centre (genesisuk.org) in Manchester has been measuring the effects of an intermittent calorie restriction diet, similar to the 5:2

diet, in women with a high risk of developing the disease.

Because excess weight is often associated with an increased risk of breast cancer, lowering weight can reduce the risk by up to 40%. But this form of dieting might offer extra benefits at cellular level.

In one study, the intermittent fasters lost nearly twice as much weight as the 'daily dieters and also showed greater improvements in 'insulin sensitivity' – which is an excellent result in terms of diabetes prevention (see more about this later in the chapter).

The BRRIDE (Breast Risk Reduction Intermittent Diet Evaluation) study has analysed breast and body tissues to see if the diet has made changes to how the genes are behaving. The hope is that that a diet of 1,800 calories five days a week, and 600 calories two days a week, may reduce the activity of the SCD gene which is thought to be a factor in the development of breast cancer.

As I've mentioned before, most of my female relatives on my mother's side of the family have had breast cancer diagnoses. Apart from my regular mammograms, I've felt powerless in the face of this history. Until now – the evidence may not yet be there in black and white but and I await the outcome of this study with particularly keen interest. Dr Michelle Harvie and her Genesis team have also written a new book summarising their dietary advice – there are full details of this, and all the research in this chapter, in the Resources section at the end of the book.

Prevention is – obviously – better than cure, but there are also indications from research in animals, and some limited studies of humans, that fasting at the right time can make chemotherapy treatment easier to tolerate, and perhaps more successful. One theory is that fasting puts the body's healthy cells into the slower-paced repair mode, but the 'rogue' cancer cells are still proliferating. So the healthy cells are less vulnerable to the toxic effects of chemotherapy, while the malignant cells which the chemo is targeting, are attacked more effectively. Further research in this area is ongoing as I write though any decisions about fasting before such treatment must be discussed with your oncology team.

Heart disease

Cardiovascular disease affects almost every family – it's the leading cause of death in the UK and the world. The term is used more broadly than you might think, to include high blood pressure, heart attacks and also strokes, so it's understandable that it's a major concern.

It's also one of the areas of medicine that researchers are focusing on when they're assessing the benefits of fasting diets.

In a range of animal studies, rodents saw a decrease in blood pressure, heart rate and cardiovascular disease risk indicators when they were put on ADF regimes. In another experiment on rats, the damage caused when a heart attack was deliberately induced was less in those being fed ADF than normal diets.

Krista Varady and her team at the University of Illinois have led the research with human subjects in this field. She's run a number of studies in the field (find more details in the resources section), which have shown that intermittent fasting is effective in helping people lose weight – and also appears to result in less loss of muscle than conventional diets. The important results for cardiovascular health were the reduction in levels of LDL (or 'bad') cholesterol and triglycerides in the blood, as did blood pressure readings in one study.

In our group of 5:2 dieters, six have already reported lower blood pressure readings and several more have seen lower levels of 'bad' cholesterol.

Type 2 diabetes

I've seen first-hand how Type 2 (or 'adult onset') diabetes is not the minor inconvenience many people assume it to be. The condition can cause cardiovascular problems, kidney disease, damage to the retina, nerve problems and damage to circulation in the legs and feet that can even lead to amputation.

Type 2 diabetes is increasing dramatically in adults right across the world, but more children and young people are being diagnosed with it, too, mainly due to the increase in obesity levels in this age group. The implications for the health of individuals – and the cost for health care – are frightening.

Type 2 diabetes develops when the body becomes less efficient at dealing with the sugars that we consume through food. When we eat, much of the food is turned into simple sugars, to provide energy to the cells. The hormone insulin, produced by the pancreas, helps to regulate blood sugar levels – too much is dangerous so insulin sends an instruction to the cells to take in more glucose, so the levels in the blood will drop.

The problem comes when the pancreas stops producing enough insulin or when the cells stop being as responsive or sensitive as they should be to the hormone. This happens most frequently in people who are overweight, because excess weight makes it harder for the body to regulate blood sugar, but can also happen in those of normal weight.

For many years, dieting wisdom has favoured 'grazing' as a way of keeping blood sugar stable. The idea is that you snack between meals, so your blood sugar levels are never allowed to drop (a drop will send hunger signals to the brain, prompting you to eat more). This idea can work if you eat healthy food in small portions – but as we've seen, the temptations to snack on high-fat and sugar foods are great. Which means you put on weight *and* your pancreas has to work overtime.

It seems to make sense to me, as a non-scientist, that reducing the number of sugar/insulin spikes you experience by eating less often during the day would make it easier to regulate blood sugar levels. It can also affect levels of fat, because insulin is **lipogenic.** While insulin is circulating, your body lays down fat stores, instead of burning fat – another reason why dieters would want to reduce too many spikes.

Which should be exactly what intermittent fasting does – if we choose to go without food, our body will turn instead to getting its energy from stored sources.

So what does the research say? Animal studies (particularly on rats) certainly suggest that fasting may have a positive effect on how they process glucose – though not all human trials show the same results. However, the Genesis cancer study outlined above found that women who followed an intermittent calorie restriction regime showed bigger improvements in their insulin sensitivity than those who followed a traditional diet.

Another study showed that fasting, without reducing the total number of calories consumed, made the body more responsive to insulin.

There is still more work to be done, but of course, simply losing body fat also reduces the risk of Type 2 diabetes. So if fasting helps you do that, it will also cut your risk, or help you control diabetes if you already have a diagnosis.

Asthma, auto-immune disorders and other chronic conditions

Numerous other studies are underway to measure the effect of intermittent fasting on conditions which affect our quality of life.

Dr James Johnson, whose book *The Alternate Day Diet* offers a version of intermittent fasting, has carried out research on people with asthma undertaking his diet, and found that 19 out of 20 people who followed it saw improvements in their symptoms.

He also studied over 500 people who've followed his Alternate Day regime – the subjects reported a range of improvements to conditions including 'insulin resistance, asthma, seasonal allergies, infectious diseases of viral, bacterial and fungal origin, autoimmune disorder (rheumatoid arthritis), osteoarthritis, symptoms due to CNS inflammatory lesions (Tourette's, Meniere's), cardiac arrhythmias (PVCs, atrial fibrillation), menopause-related hot flashes.'

That'll be hot flushes, to us in the UK. Certainly, members of our 5:2 group have seen improvements in a number of long-standing health concerns, ranging from hormonal problems like Pre-Menstrual Syndrome and Perimenopausal symptoms, through to joint inflammation and restless leg syndrome.

> *Weight is coming off, I look better in clothes and the rheumatoid arthritis in my hands doesn't hurt so much, and I have more movement in my fingers without them cracking. Will be interested to see how the blood pressure is when I see the doctor next.*
>
> ANITA, 51

> *I had some quite severe menopausal problems and whilst I did not particularly expect the diet to make any difference, it was a nice surprise to find that it does. My night sweats have stopped and whilst I get the occasional hot flush, they're not nearly as bad as they were.*
>
> SALLY, 49

Anecdotal evidence, of course, but I am sure there will be more to come as 5:2 and intermittent fasting grows in popularity.

A word on gender differences

For many years, medical research tended to assume that female bodies worked the same as male ones – so they carried out research on men and applied the findings to both.

There's more recognition now that this can lead to false conclusions, and there are specific concerns around whether women – especially during their fertile years – may not respond in the same positive ways to ADF or intermittent calorie restriction. Sleep disturbance and a reduction in fertility have been noted in both sexes but especially in females. It's not surprising – fasting is stressful to the body (though it's 'good' stress when it's controlled) so sleep may be harder and reproduction is not top priority if your body is primed to focus on survival.

It does mean that 5:2 may not be advisable if you're trying to conceive, though of course, losing weight before trying can increase your chances of a healthy pregnancy if you are overweight.

The more aware we are of the possible pros as well as cons of this diet, the better. Of course, it has to be a personal decision but there are relevant links in the resources section.

What about Starvation Mode?

Over the years, the idea of Starvation Mode has been a scary prospect for all dieters: as I said in my diary entry, friends mentioned it to me when I began this diet.

The concern is that if the body is deprived of food for a lengthy period, it will take emergency action, effectively 'rationing' the number of calories it uses and becoming so efficient in using them that if you then go back to eating normally, you will put more weight on, because your body is being over efficient.

In other words, starvation mode might have protected Stone Age Man (and woman!) from premature death – but it might also stop 21st century man and woman ever fitting into those skinny jeans …

It is hard to work out what's fact and what's fiction when it comes to this 'mode' – some diet gurus refer to it as a myth, others hold it up as the bogeyman of dieters. A human body deprived of food for a long time – 72 hours or more, though opinions vary – will begin to break down cells to produce what it needs and that's likely to mean muscle mass will decrease, the longer the starvation lasts. That's *not* a good thing.

The key words here appear to be **lengthy period** – which is the beauty of the 5:2 approach. Not only does intermittent calorie restriction help with willpower – you only have to resist temptation till you're back off the diet tomorrow – it also prevents any real risk of counter-productive changes to your metabolism because you're not restricting calories for long enough to (non-medical term here) freak your body out.

Which has to be good news for your hard-working cells – and your health overall.

Body – and mind

The research is impressive and exciting. But is that going to be enough to boost your willpower when you're craving chocolate at 4pm?

Possibly. But luckily, fasting also has powerful effects on your brain, your mood and your attitude to food. In Chapter Four, I'll explore these in much more detail.

But first, the next instalment of my diet diary. I've got one fast under my belt – now what about the rest of my life?

Kate's 5:2 Diary Part Three:

AUGUST & SEPTEMBER 2012

MyFitnessPal keeps shouting at me

Mood: excited, curious, lucky

So. One fast down, the rest of my life to go ...

The day after my first Fast Day feels amazing – and I must admit I go a bit OTT with the feasting. The TV show says you can eat pretty much what you want on your non-diet days so ... well, I behaved myself till tea-time – even cutting the portion size of my yogurt breakfast – but then it all went a bit Thank God It's Friday Night Now Let's Eat Everything in the Fridge ...

I started well, with a blueberry and yogurt breakfast at just 104 cals, then had a Panini at lunchtime. But at dinner ...

Italian Rose Wine	500 ml	300 cals
Millionaire's Shortbread Dessert		440 cals
Tortilla Chips	25 g	119 cals
Edamame, Pea and Wasabi Dip,	125 g	208 cals
Wholemeal Roll		155 cals
Garlic Mushrooms	100 g	135 cals
Cherry Tomatoes, 5 tomatoes	60 g	12 cals
Country Life Butter	10 g	69 cals
Graze Box, Toffee Apple		68 cals
	Total	**1,506 cals**

I'm a bit ashamed to post it all. There's a dessert here that almost totalled my entire calorie consumption yesterday plus nearly two-thirds of a bottle of wine (I am celebrating *not* being on a Fast Day?).

And yet … I need to be honest with myself: we all have our bad days and it still came to only a little bit more than the 1,876 I'd worked out is what I could eat without gaining any more weight.

I'm definitely not going to monitor all of my feast days, but it's almost reassuring to know that on this diet I can eat all of those rather yummy things – now and then – and still potentially lose weight if I am careful on the Fast Days. Speaking of which …

Fast Day 2 is a Saturday and I eat exactly the same as I ate on the first Fast Day. Which I thought would be boring but is actually pretty liberating. What's wrong with sticking to a breakfast option that is tasty and you know will stop you feeling ravenous?

The Schoolmarm in my computer

MyFitnessPal is quite cross with me, though. On a Fast Day, I notice that it tells me off for eating too little – saying I might go into starvation mode … luckily, all I've read about the science says that one day's fasting at a time won't affect my metabolism.

The strangest thing is that I've begun to *like* my Fast Days … even look forward to them. I feel it's a day off from thinking about food, and also a bit of a 'rest' for my body, which seems to fit in with what the programme said – that your body repairs itself while it's not running fast on protein.

I've been experimenting with eating at different times. With so much diabetes in my family, I'm interested in the effects of insulin and it strikes me that part of the benefit of fasting might be that your body isn't having to produce insulin all the time. So maybe trying to eat fewer meals a day is a good idea?

Hunger? Bring it on!

Just as strange is how hunger feels. I'd forgotten. Often what I'd mistaken for hunger is actually thirst or even boredom.

But now that I let myself get hungry on my Fast Days, it's not nearly as scary or overwhelming an experience as I feared. I'm aware that I am so lucky that I can avoid food for one or two days a week without worrying whether the food will be there when I want it to be. Eating less feels like a check-in – a reminder of what the right amount is to eat, and how fortunate we are that there will be food when we're ready.

August is party month!

I knew when I decided to embark on the diet that August wasn't going to be easy – I had lots of parties and events to go to, and so reasoned that my diet was a) going to be hard to follow and b) probably more about stopping the rot than helping me lose any weight. In total, I fast on seven days this month – and my expectations are realistic.

Weight on 31 August: 156lbs - total lost so far, 5lbs

Days on diet: 22

74

Hooray! That's a bigger loss than I was expecting. My clothes are looser, my confidence that I can lose weight this way is increasing … Could this be what I've been looking for at last?

Souped-up September

Party month over, now it's back to reality. I like autumn and I like the chance to give the diet a proper go now. The five pounds (2.3kg) I lost last month is a great start and it also feels sustainable.

I'm now settling into a routine: Fast Days are Mondays and Wednesdays, so my weekends are free for eating out and enjoying myself without calorie counting.

I'm also skipping breakfast on my Fast Days, except for black coffee. And although I am a keen cook, on Fast Days I rely on very simple foods: salads, ready-made soups, perhaps some berries or yogurt. But it also means I can plan to enjoy doing some baking at the weekends, something that was completely out of bounds when I low-carbed or calorie-counted the whole time.

But on 5:2, I'm hardly doing any calorie counting now, even on my Fast Days. I'm using MyFitnessPal sometimes, but I'm getting to know by instinct what the right level of food is.

Beetroot power

The weather changes mid-month, and I worry about switching from salads, to relying on soup. So I experiment with the chunkier ones you buy in pots in the supermarket. Even the ones with cheese or cream rarely contain more than 150 cals a portion, so they'll usually form the basis of my food for the day. I rather like that most of my food is contained in one pot: a Fast looks less daunting then somehow.

One of my choices is beetroot soup – I am surprised I haven't turned beetroot pink as my Fast Days often include some of the red peril – especially the 'sweet fire' spicy beetroot I can eat by the bucket load. Still, whatever works for me, eh?

On top of my daily soup ration, there's then room for a couple of 100 calorie snacks or treats: beetroot (!), some frozen berries with yogurt and a tiny amount of muesli for texture, a couple of apples, a banana, the world's smallest portion of tortilla chips. One evening I am meeting friends and don't want to cancel so I even allow myself a 100 calorie glass of wine. It does seem a bit decadent to be 'using' a fifth of my calories on alcohol but at least I'm a cheap date.

The doll's house portions are slightly surreal and maybe a bit sad-looking on even the smallest plates I have in the house – but because it's only a couple of days a week, I don't care. I can see how the measuring and weighing could become an obsession, and a not altogether healthy one, which is why I think the days when you eat what you like are important for psychological, as well as physiological, reasons. It's about enjoying the pleasure of food, which is so often absent in a diet.

Feasting not feeding!

I've decided to call my 'eating' days 'Feast Days' – on the TV show, they called them 'feed' days which had a slightly farmyard feel about it, and also reminded me a bit of an article I'd read about 'feeders' – men who like to date larger women and watch as they eat a lot. Those two ideas aren't really fitting in with my hopes for this lifestyle, whereas 'feast' feels far better. The point is not to indulge in a Nigella-frenzy of cakes and puddings, but to savour the food on the days when you're free to eat what you like.

I also find that the early tendency to overdo it slightly on my 'feast' days is reducing as I get used to the diet. One reason is that after counting the calories the day before, I am more aware of what everything contains – so a chocolate brownie from Costa is something I choose to savour after a small lunch, rather than something I bolt down unnoticed as I run for the train. And it tasted so good ...

The other reason is that all your senses are heightened after a day of fasting. Even a single slice of peanut butter on toast feels like a feast after a day when I've managed just fine on fewer than 500 calories ...

Weight on 30 September: 152lbs

Total lost: 9lbs, Days on Diet: 52

I slowed down a little so it's still not a dramatic weight loss, but at this rate, I should have lost a stone or more by Christmas, and be back into the healthy BMI zone.

It's a steady reduction, but it feels like a huge breakthrough, and it really is. When I remember how I felt in July – that my weight and my attitude to food were out of control, that I had no way of 'stopping the rot' – I feel very lucky.

And, of course, I'm seeing the difference. My clothes are looser and even my bra needs adjusting. Could the dreaded back fat – one of those *Daily Mail* obsessions – be facing its nemesis?

Roll on October …

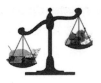

CHAPTER FOUR:

The Hunger Game – Fasting is good for the brain

Reading my diary now a few months on, it strikes me even more forcefully how important the right mental attitude is to dieting success.

Or at least, people who are successful in losing weight are those who have the mental strength to ignore cravings for long-term physical benefit. It's something I know many dieters – including myself – find difficult. If the body showed the results of that slice of chocolate cake overnight, it might be easier.

As we've established, our bodies are built to consume and conserve energy for survival. Pretty vital for early man, but in the industrialised 21st century, when many of us are lucky enough to have a vast choice and availability of food, making the 'right' choices about what we consume can be easier said than done. In theory, we have lots of appetising fresh produce available, and can make the right decisions: in practice, I know many of us feel out of control.

If you read the diary entries I've included in this book, you'll get a sense that my own weight issues result from a whole cocktail of factors:

- switching from an active job to a sedentary one;
- hating most forms of exercise;
- a sweet tooth – and a savoury one, too;
- a love of cooking, especially baking;
- a slightly addictive personality;
- a naturally, um, curvy body shape;
- a strong association between food and comfort or reward. Which means that whenever I'm feeling a bit rubbish about how tight my jeans are, my first instinct is to head straight for the biscuit tin.

What's your reason?

How about you? Why not take a couple of minutes to think about the reasons you might not be making the right choices?

Do any of these ring a bell?

- Stress – we lead busy lives, commute long distances, and work long hours: often we turn to food, particularly dishes high in fat or sugar, to provide rapid energy boosts to help us meet a deadline or comfort ourselves after a hard day.

- Commercial interests – manufacturers and retailers know that processed foods often generate higher profits, so these are marketed in ways that promote those energy boosting or comforting qualities: it's often easier to buy 'treat' foods or fast food when we're on the move than to try to buy or prepare fresher or unprocessed foods.
- Mixed messages about which foods are healthy – with some foods labelled 'low fat' turning out to be high sugar, or vice versa.
- Media images of beauty – including air-brushed photographs – present such perfect human specimens that we lose sight of what normal or healthy is – and when we can't live up to the impossible, we comfort ourselves with food.
- Upbringing – our own attitudes to food as a reward or punishment will be closely related to our upbringing and those around us – offering biscuits or alcohol to 'compensate' for doing something unpleasant, or experiencing conflict, for example.
- Hunger Phobia – we are often so busy 'grazing' or eating food throughout the day that we become terrified of feeling hungry even though for most of us in industrialised nations, it will only be a temporary state. Yet that constant feeding can also remove the anticipation that goes with building up to a delicious meal or your breakfast, say.

And finally, don't forget the fact our bodies are designed to prefer the taste of high-energy foods!

Remember how it feels to be hungry?

I had forgotten until I started this diet. I often ate because I was thirsty or bored, and had totally lost touch with the basics of appetite or enjoying the anticipation before sitting down to eat.

The first days of fasting were a revelation – because I realised I could feel hungry, acknowledge it, and then carry on with my day-to-day life. I would distract myself with sparkling water, black coffee or herbal tea, or even exercise. The pangs came in bursts and if I could ignore those, then they'd subside.

The key to being able to ignore those nagging hunger pangs? I knew it would be different the next day. I knew that if I couldn't put off eating what I fancied just for a few more hours until the next day (and knowing all the benefits to my body), then really there was no hope for me at all.

Willpower deserts me when a diet is never-ending. But when it's simply a matter of anticipating and enjoying my food the next day, it's so much easier.

Many others agree that soon the 'restriction' of a Fast Day begins to feel more like a 'liberation' from worrying about food – and allows the rest of your life to feel normal.

It allows me to have my Saturday night meal out and a few glasses of wine on a Friday without feeling as though I have 'broken my diet'. This means my relationship with my husband doesn't have to change, as we always eat out on Saturdays.

JULIE, 45

Fat crimes and punishments

The problem I've had with previous diets has been the feeling of deprivation – even punishment that constant calorie counting can provoke. You might well recognise this: you start with the best of intentions but soon feel as though your newly restricted food intake is the penalty for being greedy. Then, in a difficult moment, you think 'sod it, if I'm greedy then so be it' and console yourself with your comfort food of choice – chocolate, cheese, bread, wine – which triggers a whole new cycle of guilt …

The issue with regimes such as low-carbing, which require you to cut out most of an entire food group, is that it means you may never be able to enjoy the things you love or that form the staples of so many national diets – you see cake as sinful, or begin to fantasise about bread to go with your soup. Plus you gain a reputation as the picky one at friends' dinner parties or celebrations, which highlights the fact you're on a diet 'again' and also highlights any failures.

This diet changes how you view your eating habits – and the change is likely to be permanent. In fact, many people prefer not to call 5:2 a 'diet' at all, because of the negative associations with unworkable or abandoned weight loss regimes. I use diet here because it's brief and can also simply mean what you eat: but you may prefer to call this a plan, an approach, a way of eating or a lifestyle.

I see my Fast Days as a mini-break for my body, not to mention a break from cooking, as I tend to minimise the time in the kitchen. It's a reminder that there's more to life than food – it takes a few Fast Days to get used to that, but for me, it's liberating.

When you feel like you just HAVE to have something to eat, as hard as it may seem, just remember how bloated some foods make you, or the time you overindulged and felt bad, and remember how your body is using this 'fast' time to do really good things like healing and cleansing, and by the time you've remembered all of that you won't feel hungry again and it gets easier and easier to do.

Zoe, 38

I've talked elsewhere about how hunger is no longer something that scares me – and this diet is also teaching me to enjoy my food more on both Fast and Feast Days – my taste buds come alive and I enjoy every mouthful.

Without wishing to sound too precious, I am also more *grateful* for the food I eat. Knowing that I can eat if I really need to if the hunger becomes too great makes me feel lucky that I have that choice, when so many people don't.

The psychological benefits are one thing – but there also seem to be benefits at cellular level, in terms of brain function.

Effects on the brain: sharper, for longer?

The 'Horizon' TV programme introduced us to a rather special breed of mouse. One that had been bred to develop Alzheimer's disease. Different groups of these mice were then fed different diets – some the equivalent of junk food, others as much normal food as they wanted, and then another group were subjected to 'intermittent energy restriction' – a day on/day off regime similar to ADF.

The last group were much slower to develop Alzheimer's even though they were destined to do so. Tests showed that the mice benefited from a range of changes, including an increase in levels of BDNF, a protein that helps to protect existing neurons (brain cells) and encourage the growth of new ones. The mice on the ADF style regime also had better memories. BDNF has also been proven to have an anti-depressant effect.

Why would fasting help the brain?

But why would this be happening? Again, common sense suggests that on reduced calories, the brain would be slowing down its activity, as the cells of the body do, rather than 'wasting' energy.

Neuroscientist Mark Mattson, from the American National Institute on Aging, believes there's a biological reason why fasting would make the brain function better: if early man couldn't find or catch food, he'd go hungry and, ultimately, die. Therefore it makes absolute sense that his brain should work harder to either think up or discover new sources of food or remember where he found it the last time.

So, fasting stresses the nerve cells but – as we've seen with the other medical research – this stress may be good stress, improving mental fitness, just as exercise stresses the muscles to improve physical fitness.

The research has implications not only for Alzheimer's disease and other forms of dementia, but also strokes. Professor

Mattson is now planning more research in humans to see whether fasting can stave off age-related cognitive decline. There are indications that the greatest benefits start at middle-age, so it may be that beginning this way of eating before that stage of life has less significant results.

The practical difficulties of research into the brain – not least that changes can often only be detected in patients when an autopsy is carried out after death – mean conclusive evidence on some of these areas will take time. But Mattson himself reportedly switched from a calorie restriction diet to intermittent fasting ... like many of the experts in this field who are adopting the lifestyle with the same enthusiasm they show in their research.

Mood and energy boosts – the biggest surprise of all

I hate it when the clocks go back. I don't suffer from Seasonal Affective Disorder – the depressive symptoms many people experience during the winter months – but my mood and energy levels are definitely affected by the dark and cold. I can be a bit of an Eeyore, to put it mildly.

As I write, it's every bit as dark and cold this January as it normally is, yet I feel more energetic than I did in the summer, and almost irritatingly positive. And when I look back at my diary entries, I notice that's been an upward trend since I started the diet.

I'd assumed this was because I was feeling good about my weight loss, but even so it seemed particularly noticeable. And then I read Dr Mosley's new book, *The Fast Diet*, which offers advice based on his excellent programme, and also expands on some of the science. In it, he mentions that Mark Mattson believes this may be due to increasing levels of the BDNF protein caused by fasting.

I was fascinated and since following this up, I've read plenty more evidence, including studies that show stress can decrease BDNF levels in the brains of rats, with adverse effects on parts of the brain that are also associated with depression in animals and humans. Anti-depressant medications and even electroconvulsive therapy have been shown to reverse this decrease – so if fasting is doing the same, this could be incredibly exciting for those who have a history of depressive illness. It may also be one of the reasons experience of fasting can be so uplifting even for those who don't suffer. Interestingly, exercise can also reverse age-related declines in BDNF levels – and many of us fasting have seen our energy and inclination to exercise increase, too.

The more I read, the more the links between so many varied diseases become clear – and the more excited I am by the work scientists like Mattson, Varady and Longo are doing.

To sum up:
So – 5:2 and other intermittent fasting or restriction diets can:
- Save you money
- Help you lose weight with minimal hassle
- Make it easier to maintain a healthy weight

And they may:

- Reduce your chances of developing life-threatening diseases
- Change your attitude to food and hunger
- Help you stay mentally sharper, for longer
- Boost your mood and energy levels, often dramatically

In the next part of the book, I'll explain how to adapt this diet so it works best for you. But first, will my quest for winter sun be my diet undoing?

Kate's 5:2 Diary Part Four:

OCTOBER & NOVEMBER 2012

Hiccups in the sun

Mood: evangelical, positive, flexible

OCTOBER

Everyone I talk to seems to know someone who is doing this diet – and it's as appealing to men as to women. I've been chatting to men about why, especially as so many men I know are reluctant to admit to dieting. Is it the all or nothing nature of the Fast Days? The simplicity of it? Or maybe it's just that it *really* works?

I've also set up a group on Facebook called The 5:2 Diet so we can share our experiences. But the Facebook group is only the start – I feel so evangelical about this plan that I've decided to write all I know about it as an e-book – the book I wish there'd been when I first heard about it.

OK, I'm not a scientist, but I did work as a journalist on news, documentaries and food programmes at the BBC for fifteen years, so I'm pretty used to separating fact from fiction. Plus, I've learned a huge amount about how the diet works in real life, by talking to others who are doing it.

The hiccups

Of course, the moment I decide to write about the diet, my

weight loss stalls. I lose nothing in the first week and feel slightly disheartened. There's a second hiccup on the horizon. I'm off on holiday to Tenerife for a week this month and I know I won't be fasting there, so I decide on a pre-emptive strike, switching to ADF – fasting every other day – for the week beforehand.

Again, I'm surprised how easy it is. I simply fall into a routine of eating well but unrestrictedly one day, and then being extra careful the next. I hardly weigh any foods out any more but am grateful for supermarket fresh soups … I know how cheap it is to make your own, but it also involves being tempted to add little extras to the recipe, whereas these pots involve no more preparation than pressing a button on the microwave.

Cheap as chips

Despite buying ready-made soups, I'm saving money through this diet – in fact, I must remember to stop buying as many groceries as my freezer won't fit all the things I buy but then don't eat.

I'm cutting back on my snacking on Fast Days, but also on Feast Days because I am somehow more able to ask myself the question: do I really want this? If I do, then it's absolutely fine. But even being able to ask that question seems to curb my appetite.

And on the Fast Days I am eating very little, so my shopping bill is going down – unlike when I was low-carbing, and had to buy lots of expensive protein – or when I was doing normal calorie counting and spent a fair amount on special 'low-cal' options which always cost more.

There are occasional comedy moments, too – like the day I took a chip off my boyfriend's plate, then insisted on weighing a similar-sized one and entering it into MyFitnessPal. One chip = 8 calories = too much!

A week off fasting

Back from my hols: and I didn't count a single calorie while I was there. Buffet breakfasts, buffet dinners and lots of lovely Spanish wine.

Buffets are notoriously bad news for dieters. I've read about research that shows the variety makes us go a bit crazy, grabbing a little bit of this and that and the other which adds up to far more calories than we'd eat at a normal meal. But on the holiday, I am more conscious of stopping when I am hungry, not least because my bikini body is still not as svelte as I'd like it to be.

With that in mind I do something unprecedented – go to the hotel gym! Four times. It's not easy because the weather is hot and the gym's not air-conditioned and the equipment is pretty basic, but I do it. Everyone else in the gym is very buff and I feel a bit like the lardy girl in the corner. But maybe before long I'll be buff too?

Weight on October 31st: 150lbs: total lost 11lbs

Days on diet: 83

BMI 25.9 – which means I'm within a point of a healthy BMI

OK, it's only a loss of two pounds this month but I have had a great holiday, plus I think I am putting on muscle from the gym.

As for my goal – well, till now I haven't dared have one, but I think I'd like to be a nice round (well, not *that* round) 10 stone (63.5 kg) – or maybe 9 stone 13 (63 kg) to be in single figures.

NOVEMBER

Back to Fasting and Feasting

I loved my holiday but I am also looking forward to restarting my new routine. I like the thought it's doing me good as well as making me look better in my clothes. So after I get back, I switch from 5:2 to 4:3 and deliberately don't weigh myself in the week or so after I return from holidays because I don't want to feel down-hearted. But my jeans are still looser than they were.

My routine is pretty fixed now, but I'm experimenting with exercise. I did join the gym just before I started this lifestyle but it's become more important to me while I'm doing this – at first, I avoided exercising on a Fast Day but recently I've tried it and it's fine for me. I don't feel dizzy or wobbly at all. And the exercise just feels like part of what I want to do to look after myself more, and maximise the benefits of the diet. I also don't eat any more to compensate for the calories I've burned at the gym. Once I do an extra-long workout – using around 500 calories – and eat 470, which puts me into a strange 'minus' calories place on MyFitnessPal. And makes me feel *very* smug.

The eggs Florentine episode

The one thing with this way of eating is that it can be slightly less sociable. It's easy to schedule the diet for a couple of days a week when you have nothing planned, but 4:3 or ADF means you have to fast on Friday, Saturday or Sunday. Which are the days we often do something spontaneous.

That's what happened on Sunday. We went to my favourite cafe – Temptation in Brighton, you *have* to go if you're in town – and I'd thought, that's fine, I'll have the soup.

Then came the bombshell – they don't serve soup at weekends!

There was nothing on the menu that seemed likely to be under 500 calories. Their breakfasts are legendary, their cakes towering, and I was seriously grumpy as I ordered black coffee and braced myself to watch everyone else scoffing breakfast.

'This is very anti-social,' said the boyfriend. 'And perhaps a little obsessive. After all, it's only one day. One meal.'

I tried to think about the counter-arguments – the fact that the Fast Days do involve commitment. And yet he did have a point.

So I went and ordered the eggs Florentine: two poached eggs, spinach, sourdough toast and – this is the only unhealthy bit – lashings of sunshine yellow hollandaise sauce, vowing that I'd scrape off the sauce, even though it's my favourite bit.

And then I scoffed the lot.

At home, I looked up Hollandaise on MyFitnessPal. When I've tried to make it myself, it involved vast quantities of butter. So yes, it was high fat and very calorific. But so what if I'd gone over on one of my Fast Days? It's one day out of an entire lifetime. What this diet is doing is making me aware and informed about what I put in my body.

The eggs Florentine episode is a warning not to take it *too* seriously. To live a little.

And, guess what? I didn't actually feel hungry for the rest of the day…

Every day I write the book …

I've spent the month working on the 5:2 book. Researching the science, and talking to dozens of other people doing this, has made me even more enthusiastic about what we're all doing.

My only frustration is that I didn't discover this years ago.

Weight 30 November: 145 pounds: Total lost: 16 pounds

BMI: 24.9 – in the healthy range, hooray!

Days on Diet: 113

Well, I knew something good was happening as I've already swapped from my old baggy size 14 jeans back into the 12s, and even they feel loose. But it's lovely to see that reflected on the scales.

There's another remarkable thing I've noticed – usually when the clocks go back, it has a negative effect on my energy and my mood. It's OK, because I expect it, but I never feel that festive as the festive season approaches.

This year, I'm not feeling that at all. If anything, my energy levels are growing.

Christmas? Bring it on …

2

5:2
YOUR WAY

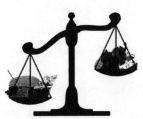

*Planning and personalising
for success*

The freedom to make fasting work for you

So you know the theory and science behind the diet – now it's time to work out what you want to achieve with this approach to eating, and to make some plans.

Unlike all the other diets I've tried over the years, 5:2 is completely flexible – you can even choose not to do 5:2 at all, but to try 4:3, 6:1 or whatever combination fits your life. It's one of the reasons it's so sustainable.

This section outlines three steps:

1. **Planning** what you want from this way of eating, and how you'll achieve it
2. **Fasting** for the first time – with lots of tips and ideas to make it as easy as possible
3. **Reviewing** what works for you – including tips on exercise, weigh-ins and Feast Days!

Step One: How much do you want to lose, and how much can you afford to eat?

Prepare for some sums. I'll keep them to a minimum, but the calculations will help you monitor your progress.

Even if you're attracted to 5:2 for health reasons, rather than weight loss, it's worth doing some measuring now, to help you see what changes it's making.

There's so much more to this than numbers, of course – it's about how you feel, and look, and how well the body's working – but if you want to fine-tune the diet, don't skip this part. The good news is that it should take you no time at all to work the figures out, and once you have, you're all set.

Goal setting: where do you want to be?

Weigh yourself
Yes, I know. If you're worried about your weight, this part is grim. But once you begin to lose weight, you'll be glad you've been honest with yourself at this stage – because your progress will be all the more impressive.

Calculate your BMI or height/waist ratio
As you read in Chapter Two, BMI isn't always the best indicator of your weight level, especially if you're very athletic, but it does give a basic indicator. You calculate it using this simple formula –

$$BMI = \text{Weight (kg)} / [\text{Height (m)} \times \text{Height (m)}]$$

Or – even more simply – by using the calculators on MyFitnessPal.com or other weight loss sites (just search for BMI calculator).

The alternative measurement I outlined in Chapter Two is your height/waist ratio, one that is increasingly seen by doctors as most useful in predicting the chance of cardiovascular problems (for an explanation, refer back to that chapter).

Measure your waist. You want the measurement to be less than half of your height. You can monitor your progress by dividing the waist size by the height – if your waist gets smaller, than so will the ratio.

As an example, here's how mine has changed before and after 5:2.

August 2012: Waist in inches (32 inches) ÷ Height in inches (64) = 0.5

January 2013: Waist (29.5) ÷ Height (64) = 0.46

You'll get the same ratio if you measure in cm. My only comment on using this as your only progress check is that it's likely to be slower to change than weight loss so may not be as immediately motivating – plus, as I've always had quite a pear shape, my starting measurement was (just) acceptable. Yet I was clearly overweight and although that measure indicates a low-ish risk of cardiovascular problems, I know my weight was putting me at higher risk of diabetes, given how common it is in my family.

So I'd suggest keeping a record of BMI, weight *and* waist measurement – and then choosing a single goal for now to focus on. You could express that as a BMI, a goal in pounds or kg, or a waist measurement ratio.

For example for me, my goal weight is **9 stone 13**, which is a) in single figures when it comes to stones, just (!) and b) represents a BMI of 23.83 …

Your goal may be less clear if you're not aiming to lose weight, but it's worth doing these, particularly if you're lean already. You don't want to slip into the underweight category as that too can have negative health implications. If you monitor your weight, you can make adjustments to how often you fast, e.g. moving from 5:2 to 6:1 with just one fasting day a week.

Diet calculations: how to reach your goal

How many days a week can you fast/calorie restrict?

The diet is called 5:2 by many people because the ratio of 5 'normal' days and 2 'diet' days works really well for most people – it offers weight loss, but it's manageable in terms of finding quieter days when it works to eat less, and also means you don't feel like you're on a diet most of the time.

But other options for weight loss include 4:3 (with 3 Fast Days) or Alternate Day Fasting (ADF). Here's a selection of how the choices our dieters have made to suit them.

Every other day – 500 calories.

SALLY, 49

I follow standard 5:2, but probably consume 7–800 calories on fast days (but I'm tall and exercise a lot).

JAMES, 43

Two days and I aim for about 600 calories a day as I don't need to lose weight.

NINA, 52

Two days. 300 calories.

SARAH, 37

Of course, the more often you fast, the faster you'll lose. For those mainly seeking the health benefits, without weight loss, 6:1 seems to be the preferred option.

How much should you eat on this diet?

Fast Days (the 2 in the 5:2 diet) are when you are restricting your calorie intake to approximately 25% of your daily calorific requirement (DCR).

I've outlined how to calculate your DCR below, because I wanted to do that myself, but since the first edition of the book, I've realised most people prefer to stick to the averages, which is much easier and works very effectively for most people.

The average active woman needs approximately 2,000 calories per day – or what we know of as calories: most food labels list kcals or kilo calories but 'calories' is used interchangeably in most diet books, including this one. So your goal intake for Fast Days is 500.

Active men need on average 2,400 calories a day so they get an extra 100 cals or a goal intake of 600 calories.

Still want to find your own precise goal? It's easy as ABC and may give you a higher goal, particularly if your BMI is very high and you have a lot of weight to lose.

Stage A: BMR

Begin by working out your Basal Metabolic Rate – how many calories someone of your size, height and age needs for survival without weight loss. That is, to keep your most basic functions going. There are two different formulas: the Harris Benedict and the Mifflin St Jeor: the latter takes age into account so that's the one I've included.

Mifflin St Jeor:
Male: BMR =
10 × weight in kg + 6.25 × height in cm – 5 × age + 5

Female: BMR =
10 × weight in kg + 6.25 × height in cm – 5 × age – 161

It's *much* easier to use an online calculator. For example, a fifty-year-old man, 5 feet 10 tall, and weighing 14 stone (196 pounds) has an estimated BMR of **1,755 calories per day**

Stage B: factor in your activity level

The BMR sounds low – so now we factor in how active you are, to give a truer estimate of your actual Daily Calorie Requirements.

Little/no exercise:
BMR x 1.2 = Total Calorie Need

Light exercise:
BMR x 1.375 = Total Calorie Need

Moderate exercise (3–5 days/wk):
BMR x 1.55 = Total Calorie Need

Very active (6–7 days/wk):
BMR x 1.725 = Total Calorie Need

Extra active (very active & physical job):
BMR x 1.9 = Total Calorie Need

You can use online calculators for this too, but it's a simple calculation. Our male dieter takes limited light exercise, so we multiply his BMR by 1.375: = **DCR of 2,413 calories**

Stage C: Lower, lower!

So to maintain his weight, our male dieter could eat up to 2,413 calories. But he's fasting to lose weight and for the health benefits, so on Fast Days he needs to eat a quarter of his DCR.

2,413 ÷ 4 = **603 calories**

Is it worth it?

So … After all those sums, we've ended up very close to the 600 average goal for men. It's up to you whether you want to do this yourself – as I say, if you're heavier, you may find this gives you a few extra calories to play with. In my case, as I record in my diary, I 'lost' 30 calories as my goal was 469 – but I suspect my weight loss would have been pretty much the same had I aimed at 500.

If you make these calculations and then lose a lot of weight, you'd want to recalculate, as your calorie requirement decreases as your weight does – UNLESS you step up your levels of activity, which may well happen as you find you have more energy and confidence.

The sums are finished. Time to tailor the diet to suit you!

Which day(s) do I fast?

Picking the right days will improve your chances of success.

The first time(s) you fast, you're likely to feel hungry at first, with possible other side-effects like headaches, or feeling cold or slightly light-headed. Most of us become used to this very quickly, but it makes sense to schedule your first couple of Fast Days for days when you have fewer commitments and can afford to take it a little easier.

Though it's best not to clear your diary completely – most of us have found that staying busy is the best distraction from any hunger pangs.

Choose days when you have no food-based social events, or don't have to be around people who might be sceptical or try to persuade you to give up. If you are responsible for family meals, then try to build in days when the meal is healthier and you can have a small portion without attracting too much fuss. I like to do my Fast Days when my partner is working late or socialising with friends because that way I won't be tempted to eat what he's eating at home!

It can be useful to have regular days e.g. Monday and Wednesday, because you can schedule around them. At first, I didn't exercise on Fast Days so scheduled around that. But it's your diet – feel free to experiment.

I definitely find it helps to mark the Fast Days on my e-calendar and to-do lists – this way I feel that I have committed to them!

If a 'whole day' fast doesn't work for you, some people fast for part-days, but still for twenty-four hours. So you might eat a normal lunch on Monday, then stick to 500 or 600 calories until a later lunch or early supper on Tuesday evening.

When do I eat on my Fast Days?

You can choose to eat your calorie allowance in one, two or even three meals, although evidence suggests that the health benefits may be higher if you restrict to two or one meals, with as little snacking as possible.

This is how Krista Varady's study worked, with participants having a single, larger meal at lunchtime on their 'fast' days. It makes sense to me because it appears to give the body less to 'do' in terms of digesting food, producing insulin etc. Dr Mosley, by contrast, decided that he would eat two meals and it still worked for him, both in terms of weight loss and reduction in IGF-1.

At the start, I could never have imagined a whole day without any food. But five months in, I frequently eat only in the early evening on a Fast Day, to try to maximise the health benefits, and I don't find it difficult at all.

Equally, if it's cold and I want some soup at lunchtime to warm myself up, I don't worry too much. And neither should you if you want to have three meals. You're still doing something great for your body.

That's the beauty of this diet compared to all the others I've tried (and abandoned): you decide how to make the diet fit your life, rather than the diet dictating how to live it. Here are how some other dieters divide up their Fast Day calorie allowances.

No breakfast. Porridge midday. Veg soup in evening. Couple of barley cups during day and perhaps a rice cake.

STEPHEN, 47

One meal in the evening with my family. Portions small except for green salad/veg. An entire bag of salad is circa 40 calories (a single egg is circa 80 calories and as for cheese or, god forbid mayonnaise…!)

MYFANWY, 49

I can't do just one meal a day as I need the psychological feeling of having three meals a day.

NINA, 52

Minding the gap

There's another way to try to maximise the health benefits – and that's by being aware of the gap between the last meal Feast Day and the first on Fast Day. And then doing the same when it's Feast Day again. I do this, as it seems to make sense to increase fasting time. For example:

Monday Feast Day:
Eat dinner at 6pm

Tuesday Fast Day:
Eat main meal at 6pm (no breakfast or lunch)

Wednesday Feast Day:
Skip breakfast, eat lunch late e.g. 2pm

Some 5:2 dieters do go for a 'full' fast, where you only drink water or herbal teas. If the 'gap' planning above is taken into account, you could fast completely for 44 hours, but there would only be one day where you don't eat.

Monday Feast Day:
Eat dinner at 6pm

Tuesday Fast Day:
Fast completely

Wednesday Feast Day:
Skip breakfast, eat lunch late e.g. 2pm

Bear in mind that total fasts can be harder to stick to, but there are many alternatives, such as compressing your mealtimes into a small 'window of eating', so you avoid food for twenty hours and limit eating to between, say, 1pm and 5pm. Again, this may maximise the benefits.

> *I try to postpone eating all day so I can eat in the evenings but I'm not sure this helps much. It probably does re: the metabolic changes needed for fat mobilisation and brain growth, because the longer we go, the better it is, but it might undermine the repair at night side of things. The research suggested eating at mid-day but I fear once I start eating I would want more.*
>
> LINDA, 52

The truth is that there isn't a study I've found comparing different fasting configurations. I am sure that will come, but in the meantime, experiment to find *your* best approach.

Consecutive or non-consecutive?

Most people schedule the days non-consecutively as the hunger pangs can be stronger and a two-day fast can become an ordeal rather than a 'mini-break'. This risks making it less sustainable than the non-consecutive option. Some doctors would also be wary of someone undertaking a fast for more than twenty-four hours without being checked thoroughly beforehand, and maybe being supervised.

WHAT will I eat on my Fast Day?

Exactly what you like ... so long as it doesn't exceed your calorie limit.

500 or 600 calories isn't a lot to play with. But, take it from me, you *can* still make satisfying choices.

> *Banana for breakfast. Apple and yogurt for lunch. Chicken and salad for dinner.*
>
> KARL, 49

> *Loads of cups of tea with a little milk, nothing till supper, then a normal family supper with few/no carbs.*
>
> JULIA, 50

> *Only water!*
>
> ROB, 42

> *All home-made food so it's hard to work out the calories. I'll avoid carbs and alcohol and have a small helping of chicken or fish and lots of vegetables – a bowl of home-made soup and fruit for the other meal. I'm aiming to only eat between 12 and 6, too, on most other days.*
>
> LINDA, 52

> *I stick to fruit and veg, beans on toast, soups, Weightwatchers ready meals.*
>
> JANE, 49

There are plenty more sample menus and food ideas in the third section of the book. I do recommend planning in advance – the very last thing you want to be doing on your first Fast Day is going into the supermarket …

Obviously, it also depends on how many meals you're planning to have – it's very easy to find ready-meals with 400–500 calories if you're only having a single meal, but it gets slightly harder if you want two or even three. That's where soups come into play – they tend to fill you up for longer, with fewer calories.

I am also more careful to remember to take a multi-vitamin during the fasts: not because I think a day or two of eating less will do serious damage, but it's a good insurance policy.

HOW will I monitor what I eat on Fast Days?

Studies suggest that dieters who keep a record of what they eat tend to be more successful, and it will help you pinpoint where you might be going wrong if you need to amend your habits or consumption. You can either do that electronically, or jot it down in a notebook.

The brilliant thing about 5:2 is that most of us only need to record what we eat on Fast Days – so much less hassle. If you're eating ready-made meals, recording your consumption can be very easy. They all have the nutritional information on the packet or just scan the barcode if you have MyFitnessPal on your phone. Online sites allow you to keep your diary completely private or, if you find it helps to keep you motivated, share it with others.

If you're cooking from scratch, weigh the ingredients carefully and then either use a calorie counter book or MyFitnessPal to add up. I prefer the latter because it does the sums for you *and* thousands of other users are constantly updating the site with new foods or brands. On top of this, you can use it to calorie-count your own recipes. It's how I've done the dishes in Part Three, for example. A digital scale is most accurate, or you could try measuring cups or spoons (so long as you don't overload them!).

At first, you'll probably be astonished at how many calories some foods contain, but you'll become used to the portion sizes you're allowed on Fast Days and it'll be second nature.

That's enough theory ... are you ready to try your first fast?

Step Two: Your First Fast

Time for lift off – and weight off!

The last section has prepared you so you know what and when to eat. So this section is mainly about strategies and tips from those of us who have been there ...

Motivation

The first Fast Day can be a rollercoaster, though most of us found it way easier than we expected. The biggest motivation for many of us has been the mantra:

It's only a day – tomorrow you can eat what you feel like!

Keeping busy is really important, as is reminding yourself of why you're doing this. Re-reading Chapters Three and Four about the potential health benefits can be really effective – and joining in with a forum (or even lurking and reading what others are saying) will make you feel you're in great company.

A checklist of practical tips

On a practical level, there are many simple things you can try that will help you stay on track.

- If you can, avoid situations where you have to watch other people eat – or have to cook for the family. If you can't get out of doing the cooking, choose Fast Days to cook the things you really don't like and they do!
- Evenings can be a dangerous time for snackers – a hobby that uses your hands (quiet at the back!) like knitting, sewing, even jigsaws, can keep you from raiding the biscuit barrel when you're watching TV.
- Don't forget to drink water! As well as eating up to your goal calorie limit, you can (and should) drink plenty of water – there's evidence that good hydration helps with fat loss. Hot water is surprisingly easy to drink, too, in winter.
- I like to drink sparkling water on Fast Days – somehow it's more enjoyable.

- Sugar-free chewing gum is another standby!
- You may also drink black coffee or tea, herb teas and diet drinks, although artificially sweetened drinks may still affect your blood sugar or insulin levels, which is not ideal on a Fast Day. There is also some debate about the effect that caffeine has on insulin – with some studies showing an increase in insulin sensitivity (which would be broadly good news) and others showing insulin spikes (less good news). As an espresso addict, I am sticking with my daily fixes for now but as with all the decisions here, it's about personal choice.
- You may feel like going to bed early on the first few Fast Days – so use it as an excuse to relax!

And **REMEMBER:**
Tomorrow you can eat what you like!

Friends and frenemies:

One question which does crop up is, *Who should I tell?*

One advantage of telling people may be increased support from family members or friends, especially if they're following the diet themselves. It may also help you stay committed if people are asking you how it's going.

However, reactions aren't always positive.

I find it embarrassing being on a fasting diet (because I know people will exclaim 'you're too thin to be doing it') so I don't talk about it outside our family. If I'm ever with other people on fasting days I tend to try and eat as little as possible without people noticing.

SARAH, 37

I told a few people I was starting the fast and it both helped & hindered me. It helped because when I was a little cranky on those first couple of fasts they just took it as the diet, but it hindered because any conversation I had where we didn't agree (not an argument, just work related or otherwise) they said I wasn't being rational because I 'needed to eat something' which wasn't the case as both times I had just eaten and they were not 'fast' days! Be prepared for doubters as most people are 'brainwashed' about 'skipping meals' and 'breakfast is the most important meal of the day' and 'your metabolism will slow down' so I don't talk about the diet any more, I just get on with it.

ZOE, 38

Men in particular can find it embarrassing to be on an obvious diet – one recent survey suggested one in three male dieters wouldn't admit it, even to their closest friends or family.

You may also worry about the impression a fasting diet might give to younger people in your family, especially now there's so much more awareness around eating disorders.

I have three daughters and I am concerned about setting a good example, and not making them too faddy.

*So when they're around I stick to something simple, like
beans on toast, which doesn't look like a 'fasting' meal.*

MARY, 50

Group therapy

An alternative to relying on friends or family is to form your
own support group or join one online. Our group of software
company employees have definitely seen the benefits of sharing:

*If a group of you are doing it, it really helps – especially
if you all do it on the same day.*

ANDREW, 42

Lots of couples are deciding to embark on the plan together
– or often, one will notice how well their partner is doing
and join in (that's actually happened to me!). A little healthy
competition can make the process more interesting.

*It helps a lot that my husband is also following it
primarily for health reasons as he doesn't need to lose
any more weight and is now having to try to eat a bit
more on 'normal' days to keep his weight from dropping
further! Lucky him ...*

ELAINE, 52

Even if you can't or don't want to get colleagues or family
members involved, the internet makes it really easy to connect
with diet soul mates. Joining in with a forum can really help
– because we can talk online to people who have been there

and ask questions without feeling embarrassed: our Facebook group grew from a handful to over 700 contributors and as a result we moved to a separate forum, at www.the5-2dietbook. com – and there are plenty more listed in the Resources section of this book.

The possible side-effects

You may not experience any of these, but here are some of the more common things dieters have experienced in the early days. Jeanny is typical:

> *I have been feeling light headed and dizzy, but I'm not sure whether it is the diet as I haven't been doing it very long yet. Also, have had several headaches.*
>
> JEANNY, 53

Unwelcome effects

Anyone who has made a change to their eating habits will know that the body can take a while to adapt – and 5:2 is no exception.

Most of us have been how surprised at how quickly we adapt to what seems like a huge change, but even so, you may experience some symptoms at first. Most are minor, but do remember that if there's anything that seems extreme or worries you, you should contact your GP.

The main effects seem to be headaches, sleep disruption and feeling the cold more in winter.

Headaches

These seem to be the number one symptom for people starting any new diet, and can be caused by a variety of factors, including dehydration (much of our water consumption comes from food, so if we eat less of it, we may get thirsty), changes to blood sugar levels, or caffeine withdrawal. The blood sugar should stabilise, and we advise drinking lots of liquids to avoid dehydration. In terms of caffeine, there's no need to cut out coffee or tea, and in fact, I'd advise against doing this at a time when you're already trying something new. Just remember to count calories if you add milk or sweeteners – or train yourself to take your coffee black.

Most people find headaches are reduced or eliminated after the first fast or two. If they continue, you can try varying meal times to cope with any blood sugar issues.

Sleep Disturbance

Some people do find it hard to sleep when they haven't eaten as much – and the mild stress that fasting causes can make you feel a little more 'hyper' than usual. I chose to see this as a welcome energy boost while it lasted, but the usual advice about sleeplessness – take a long bath before bed, read rather than watch TV, try a milky drink – might be useful. A new suggestion involves eating one or two kiwi fruits an hour before going to bed – they've been proven to improve sleep quality by up to 40%.

Feeling cold

I began the diet in August and didn't notice this, but winter starters have found that they can feel cold on Fast Days. Hot drinks and eating soup will help warm you up. You can also add spices to foods, e.g. flaked chilli goes well with soups or baked beans. Also, ginger flavours in tea can give you a nice glow. It *will* get easier.

Other effects reported by group members:

- **Irritability:** feeling hungry may make you grumpy to begin with, though hunger pangs tend to disappear rather than get worse if you ignore the sensation. Low blood sugar might also make you snappy at first though again, this should stabilise. Try one of the lower-calorie treats in the food section – it's better to do without them in the long term, but when you're starting out, be kind to yourself!
- **Digestive changes:** constipation and reflux have been reported. It's worth including fibre (e.g. baked beans) or 'digestive transit' yogurts in your Fast Days. One of our dieters was advised by her surgery nurse to ask the pharmacist about gentle laxatives, though obviously these are not recommended for anything other than occasional use.
- **Cramps:** I used to get these all the time in the first few days on low-carb diets and haven't on this one. But I know some people have and I've read about good responses to potassium, magnesium or calcium supplements.

The positives about Fast Days

Here's a list of things to remind yourself if you're wavering.

- You're doing something good for your health and your body
- You can work past hunger – it comes in waves, so make it a challenge to see how long it takes to feel better.
- It's incredibly beneficial to learn the difference between hunger, and thirst or boredom, which can become confused over time.
- You are making this choice – which tends to make you so much more appreciative of the fact that when the fast is over you can eat what you like
- Not to mention the fact that any food you do have scheduled will be savoured all the more!
- It can be a break for your mind *and* body as you focus on things other than food – though that may not kick in till you've done a few fasts

Finally, here are some tips from our 'expert' dieters.

Have a plan and measure out what 500 calories looks like. This will stop you obsessing about food ALL day long. Thinking of what you will reward yourself with is also good. I plan to have a nice Thai meal with all those 'naughty' carbs.

Zoe, 38

Try to leave breakfast as late as possible. When you eat in the morning it makes you feel like you want to eat more. I prefer to leave my meals as late as I can. For snacking, try cherry tomatoes or carrots. Not many calories but filling. I prefer getting the fast days over and done early in the week – Mondays and Wednesdays. Fasting on days when you are not at work is harder as you have more temptations around.

SUNIL, 34

Find something to keep you busy well away from food (I fast on work days, if I can; hardly have time to eat there anyway) and treat yourself on non-fasting days so you don't feel deprived.

MYFANWY, 49

Drink lots of boiled water or herbal teas on your fasting day. You'll find the flavour makes you feel as if you've eaten something. Also, if you like milk in your tea or coffee first thing in the morning and last thing at night, have it, even on fasting day. It will make you feel less as if you're being punished for something. It also helps to choose one treat that you intend to have the next day when you can eat what you want again, whether it's a bit of cake, some chocolate, a glass of wine, or a full English breakfast.

SALLY, 49

Finally, I love this cautionary tale from Myfanwy:

DON'T go food shopping on a Fast Day – last time
I did I came home with a turkey (on special offer).
Admittedly it was a runt of a turkey but I don't even
like turkey and I've never cooked one before in my life.
The family thought it was hilarious.

MYFANWY, 49

Ready, steady, fast ...
And that's all there is to it.

By the end of today, you'll have finished your first fast – the
first, we hope, of many that will help you keep a check on your
eating and improve your health.

Step Three: Review, Revise, Revitalise

The day after

You did it! And today you can enjoy the foods you love –
perhaps some of the things you were craving yesterday ...
what are you most looking forward to? We've talked a lot
about Fast Days – but what about Feast Days? These are
times to relax and enjoy food and all the great things around
food – being with friends and family, savouring the tastes and
smells and pleasure of cooking or eating out. In fact, it's not
just about the food.

I find that I sleep much deeper on starving nights and
wake up feeling more fresh than normal. Also, the sun

seems brighter, the sky bluer and the song of birds more beautiful on the day after starving. ;)

SUNIL, 34

On Feast Days you can eat 'normally' – but what does that actually mean? One of the things I've discovered since starting this lifestyle is that I did eat much more than I realised. So while my own 'doll's house portions' on Fast Days seem ludicrously small, the portions served in restaurants now often seem obscenely super-sized.

For me, the view of what a 'portion' of food is has become skewed and that's one of the reasons many of us have suffered weight problems. So, although you can eat all the things you love on your normal days, there's clearly a sensible balance. This diet will probably re-educate you by stealth. You'll become fuller sooner, and you'll enjoy your favourite foods but perhaps not in the same quantities. It won't happen overnight but most of us who're doing this long-term have noticed the effect. It's almost like a reset button on an electronic appliance that's gone haywire – fasting has made me work properly again, still enjoying food, but eating what I need and no more.

If you are aiming to lose weight, you'll still need that calorie deficit we discussed in Chapter Two: but the reset effect means **most people don't need to calorie count on Feast Days to achieve that.**

The work done by Krista Varady at the University of Illinois compared alternate day fasters who ate a low-fat diet on their feast day, with those who ate a 'normal' high-fat diet when they weren't fasting. Surprisingly – and happily – the reduction in weight and cholesterol was as good, if not better, in those participants who were encouraged to eat all their favourite dishes, including pizza and burgers.

'Rebound' eating or over-compensation simply didn't happen on the feast days.

It's a finding backed up by the software engineers who've clubbed together to track their experiences on 5:2.

> *We have seen no difference in effect if you eat high fat or low fat food on non-fasting days. In fact, where some of us have been away on holiday, we have temporarily stopped and then restarted with little overall effect.*
>
> ANDREW, 42

Of course, what you eat is one thing. How much is another matter. I admit that in the first week or two, I was tempted to over-eat the things I loved. But that soon wore off, as it has for other 5:2 dieters. Even eating your Daily Calorie Requirement (DCR) – just under 2,000 calories in my case – feels like such a feast compared to the fasting that you probably won't feel the need to exceed it and, on many occasions, you'll eat less than you used to.

Mindful eating

One tip while you're adapting would be to use the same tactic many of us use on the Fast Days – to eat very slowly, with no other distractions. So, no TV, work or multi-tasking. Savouring your food rather than throwing it down means you'll probably be less tempted to overeat. But you certainly don't need to record what you're eating on the Feast Days.

Mindfulness – a form of meditation – can be a very useful tool in both controlling appetite and feeling positive and calm about the changes you're making. A friend recommended the getsomeheadspace.com site, which offers a free introductory trial of meditations, as well as some really useful downloads, including one on mindful eating. There are also links in the resources section to interesting articles in the *Independent* and the *New York Times* about this.

What if I'm not losing enough weight?

If you have lost weight but it's slowed down, you could consider increasing from 5:2 to 4:3 or ADF to speed things along.

But if you've not lost anything a few weeks down the line, it's worth using MyFitnessPal or a calorie counting book to double-check your calorie consumption on a typical Feast Days. Obviously, as we saw in Chapter Two, fasting will cut anything from 3,000 to 6,000 calories from your weekly consumption, but if you do find you are bingeing or over-compensating, then the weight loss could be slow.

The good news is that most people find the Fast and Feast pattern helps them find a natural balance of enjoying food without overindulging. If someone had told me that at the beginning, I'd have been sceptical, but it really does happen.

It gets easier!

If you find your Fast Day tough, then take comfort from the fact that most of us have found they get easier – *much* easier. Many dieters look forward to Fast Days as they love the feeling of lightness and euphoria – feeling good physically, but also psychologically, knowing that you're doing something good for your body.

Reviewing and planning your next Fasts

The first few weeks are about experimenting with what works for you – the best mealtimes, the most satisfying foods, plus any hints to reduce any side-effects you might be feeling.

Get into the habit of planning the days you'll be fasting the next week, and preparing by buying any ready meals, or the ingredients for home-made dishes. Check the food section of this book for lots of ideas.

One thing to consider is whether you're someone who craves variety or a person who will be happy with the same foods on your Fast Day? I've mentioned my huge beetroot-fest that lasted for about a month during the diet, without any side effects. Then gradually, and naturally, I switched to something else.

If the idea of eating the same thing on Fast Days will damage your motivation, then experiment and go onto forums to check out what ideas people have, especially for eating seasonally (which is also likely to be cheaper).

Exercise and 5:2

Many people avoid vigorous exercise at first during Fast Days – until they've discovered how their bodies react to the calorie restriction.

I started doing my gym visits on Fast Days about a month after I began the diet. At first, I did feel light-headed at times, and reduced the pace a little, but I've found that I can now keep up the same exercise intensity on Fast and Feast Days.

One thing to note if you do exercise – don't eat extra on Fast Days to compensate for the calories burned.

I typically jog 6km 4 times a week. It makes no different if that is a diet day.

STEPHEN, 47

On fasting days I do thirty minutes on the treadmill at 2mph. As I have arthritis at the moment this is the most I can do without bringing on an 'episode' of arthritis, but I hope to build it up as I lose weight/get fitter. I try to do this every day but if I feel sore I will rest for a day or two.

SALLY, 49

I haven't found it easy to exercise on Fast Days, but on other days I will spend two to three evenings a week in the gym doing weights, cardio and swimming.

CLAIRE, 43

I've maintained my usual routine of daily exercise (mostly cycling to work). I generally avoid tough workouts on fasting days.

JAMES, 43

I run about four times a week – thirty mins each time. It doesn't really matter if I do it on Fast or Non Fast Days because it doesn't increase my appetite. I don't factor it into my calorie restriction because I don't think it makes that much difference.

SARAH, 37

There's a debate about whether exercising on Fast Days, or on an empty stomach before breakfast, for example, might have benefits (bit.ly/Tv2owD) although an analysis (bit.ly/Vgv6Uh) on the NHS website suggests that it's too early to draw conclusions. For now it's good to do what feels right for you but do be wary of pushing yourself too hard at first, and consult your doctor if you have any doubts at all.

Weighing in

Most diets recommend weighing yourself no more than once a week, because fluid levels and weight fluctuates so much, especially, for women, during the monthly menstrual cycle. But Dr Mosley has suggested daily weigh-ins as a tool for monitoring progress.

One of the first dieters in the Facebook group, Linda, has produced an amazing graph recording her weight every non-

Fast day since she began , which she's kindly allowed me to reproduce. The graph, shown below, shows the passage of time and it illustrates those variations very graphically – as well as showing the overall downward trend (we've kept the exact weights off – as Linda says, 'a lady has to keep SOME secrets;)'

weight

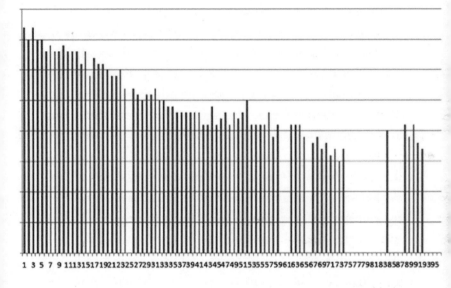

Linda explains how the graph has helped – and occasionally hindered – her.

There is quite a lot of variation from day to day. There are lots of reasons for the daily fluctuation; loss of water on fasting days due to depletion of stored glycogen; less gut content, fluid levels in the body, etc, as well as weight loss. In fact, fat loss will account

*for very little of the daily weight loss and is easily
disguised by variations in stored glycogen and gut
content. I also hit a period where food was going in
but not much was coming out (to put it delicately)
and there's a period there where I didn't fast because I
had a cold and couldn't face it, and Xmas, of course.*

Linda has fasted 32 times with a 500 calorie limit – which adds up to a calorie deficit overall of 48,000 calories, which should equate to a loss of almost 14 pounds in total. In fact, she's lost more, possibly because her DCR is a bit higher than average, so potentially she could have eaten slightly more on Fast Days.

For her (and for us!), keeping such a detailed record has been enlightening. But she also advises:

*Please don't be despondent and give up if you weigh
yourself after a fast or a week where you have been 'good'
and don't see as much of a loss as you might expect.*

The risk of despondency is the reason I don't weigh myself every day. To me, it would be a rollercoaster, even though I know there are good reasons for fluctuation. Sally feels the same:

*I was tempted to weigh myself every day (and did!)
when I started, but it can be a bit soul destroying as
you'll find you'll lose weight on fasting days then appear
to put it back on again on feasting days. It's best to
weigh once a week.*

SALLY, 49

It may be a generalisation, but I suspect that daily weigh-ins may suit men better, as they like to know where they are and may be less likely to have an emotional reaction!

If you can bear it, weigh every day, fast and non-fast, because you can track what's happening and the pattern of losing weight. Provided you stick to it, it'll still be downwards …

Kevin, 40

However often you decide to do it, record the figure in a notebook or on a site like MyFitnessPal (which will later produce a graph for you, hopefully showing your excellent progress!).

In terms of which day, or time of day, I tend to weigh the morning after the second Fast Day of a week, first thing, before I've eaten. At first it felt like cheating but so long as you always do it at the same time, then the progress or otherwise will become clear.

Rewarding yourself

Any lifestyle change can be tricky, and it makes sense to find ways to reward yourself in ways that don't involve food – the standard advice is things like a long hot bath, a massage, new clothes.

But if you're not into girly (or manly) treats, or you haven't reached your goal weight, brainstorm other rewards – a new DVD box set or even a fitness DVD; a great novel; tickets for a gig or a gallery; whatever you love doing that you don't always give yourself time to enjoy.

You could put aside the money you're saving from your grocery bill to pay for the treats.

I have even been known to reward myself with a new recipe book, for the days when I can enjoy cooking without feeling guilty. There's pleasure in the gloriously illogical knowledge that weight loss is contributing to my next delicious meal on a Feast Day!

The gift of food

I'd like to share one story from forty-three-year-old Jenny, who is finding that her fasts are making her see the world differently, too.

It really is a very good way of eating (I don't call it a diet!) and have to say, on a vaguely hippy level, I feel humbled by the fact that I can choose to go hungry. A homeless girl stopped me in the street the other day and asked if I could spare her a pound for a hot drink. I've never been approached directly like that before. But something in my brain pinged and I realised that I had chosen not to nip out of the office for a sarnie and pot of fruit since it was a fasting day. So I gave her the fiver I'd have spent on lunch. You'd think I'd given a wheelbarrow full of treasure. It's funny how things strike you at just the right time – homeless people are a factor in any big town or city yet being approached by that girl seems like proper synchronicity.

Inspired by Jenny, I made a donation to Shelter and will do the same when I hit weight loss milestones. If it's something that appeals to you, you might consider doing the same.

The best reward – it works …

Of course, you should soon begin seeing the results of the diet itself – which is the biggest reward.

Many of us see changes from week one – in January 2013, the Facebook group has had members who've lost six pounds in a week, while others haven't lost anything until the second or third weeks. My own weight loss was very undramatic but it felt sustainable and what kept me going was the knowledge that the health benefits were the most important thing to me.

Trouble-shooting

Most people who embark on the diet find it sustainable and simple. But what if it's *not* working quite as well as you'd hoped?

- Review your Feast Days – do a trial calorie count on one or two days. If it exceeds your DCR by a large amount you may need to adjust your portion sizes. The good thing about having fasted is that cutting back slightly should be very easy.

- There are a few people who stick to the diet but don't see the results. If you've done some calorie counting and you're not bingeing, it may be worth talking to your doctor about thyroid or other issues, especially if you've struggled on other diets too.

Now move on to Part Three – it's all about the food!

3

EATING THE

5:2

WAY

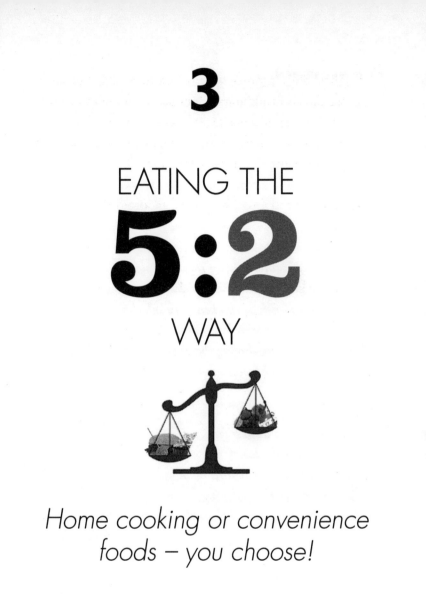

Home cooking or convenience foods – you choose!

For starters...

There's no point in fibbing about this – you can't eat much on your Fast Days. But even 500–600 calories can fill you up, and for most of us, it's far less daunting than a 'true' fast where you'd eat nothing at all.

The way people structure their Fast Days varies – there's no right answer!

Usually have 100g frozen fruit for breakfast (thawed – 29 cals). Weight Watchers tomato soup (76 cals) at lunchtime and either a Weight Watchers frozen meal in the evening, or fish or chicken with salad in the evening to make up to the 500, less if possible. Allow 60 cals for 2 coffees with milk during the day. Weight Watchers chicken and beef hotpots are about 230 cals each.

STEPH, 49

1 x coffee (white with sugar)
1 x cup-a-soup for lunch
2 pieces of fruit in late afternoon
A decent meal in the evening
Also drink herbal teas during the day if I feel peckish

SUNIL, 34

Shop-bought soups (as low-calorie as possible) and ready meals, with some veg and fruit. I aim for 500 calories and total it as I go.

VAL, 56

Oats So Simple Porridge with Semi-Skimmed Milk at around 1pm (180 calories)

Bachelors Golden Vegetable Cup-a-soup at around 4:30pm (59 calories)

Dinner usually around 300–350 calories, often from the Hairy Bikers Diet Cook Book which is excellent as it's not low fat and gives calories per portion.

ANDREW, 42

I've started making dhal, baked beans are good, salads are filling, make my own tom soup with a half stock cube in a little boiling water, 1/3rd tom puree added once that's dissolved, herbs and garlic puree added (the stuff in the tube), then topped up with more boiling water. Easy. I avoid hi GI foods.

LINDA, 52

Yogurt, cuppa soup, and an omelette!

GRAEME, 38

As I outlined in Step Two, you will need to make decisions about how often you eat on your Fast Day – one, two, or three meals – and also whether you want to cook, or use ready-made meals. Many of us do both, though as I carry on with this regime I veer more towards spending the minimum time in the kitchen. I adore cooking but it's less fun when you're measuring every teaspoon of vinegar, or fretting over lemon juice.

In this part of the book, I will make suggestions for ready-made *and* home-made options for breakfasts, lunches and dinners, plus snacks, treats and tips for eating out. Equally, if you want to munch on muesli at tea time, or sip soup for breakfast, it's your call!

The recipes are pretty simple – and do please adjust them as you wish. Or you can put your own dishes into the Recipe section of the www.MyFitnessPal.com site to work out how many calories your favourites contain. You can make a huge batch of soup or stew and then measure it out into portions to freeze – this way you enjoy all the economic benefits of a home-made dish, but run less risk of accidentally going over the limit for the day.

I'm a vegetarian and I do recommend focusing on fruit and veg on your Fast Days as you'll get more for your calories – though there are meaty suggestions too.

Also bear in mind that some scientists say eating a lot of protein may switch on IGF-1 which may be counter-productive. Dr Mosley has said he keeps protein down to under 60g on Fast Days – as an example, a medium egg contains approximately 7g and 100g of cooked chicken breast contains around 30g. You may prefer to do the same – it's a balancing act, though, as protein tends to keep you full for longer.

I've included an **A–Z of Ingredient Inspiration** (with a few letters missing, I must admit – ever tried finding a nice food beginning with U?) to give you new ideas for seasonal produce. Plus there's a list of **sweet and savoury snack ideas**, for those times when you *need something now*!

Finally, I've included a section of **daily menu ideas** to help you get started – plus a template so you can plan your own.

A note on measurements: I am a confused cook – I weigh myself in pounds, measure myself in feet and inches, but cook in grams, especially since 5:2 because the measurements seem more precise. I hope this doesn't make things too confusing – there are links to conversion charts in the Resources section.

Food and Fasting tips

Before we get to the recipe section, here are some helpful guidelines which should help on Fast Days.

Measure, measure, measure (at least till you get used to it!)

Yes, it's a bit tedious but it can also be very enlightening. It will really give you an insight into why we might be consuming more calories than we ever realised before. Weighing and then recording *exactly* what you're eating on the Fast Days – right down to a teaspoon of balsamic vinegar or a sprinkling of sunflower seeds – is the best way to avoid the temptation to cheat. Of course, once you're more used to the quantities you can eat on Fast Days, you won't need to measure so frequently.

Doll's house meals

The simplest approach to doing this diet is cut out all snacks, and then measure tiny portions of the foods you and your family normally eat (checking the calorie counts carefully until you can estimate them). Sometimes it's easier than cooking something entirely separate when time is short.

It helps to use smaller plates or dishes – I think of my Fast Day yogurt and fruit as a doll's-house-sized portion.

Vitamin 'insurance'

It makes sense to take a multi-vitamin during the fasts, just to make sure you're getting enough nutrients. Of course, if you're eating lots of vegetables, you might be getting even higher levels of certain vitamins than usual, but I think taking a good multi-vitamin is a sensible move for anyone who is dieting.

Meal replacement shakes and bars

There's no need to buy 'special' foods for your Fast Days, and personally I prefer to eat foods that are similar to what I eat on normal days – just smaller portions or with fewer 'naughty' additions.

Having said this, diet shakes, soups and bars have proved useful for some people – they are fortified with vitamins, and they also offer very precise calorie-controlled portions, so you know exactly what you're getting.

Although the milkshakes were boring, I can see the benefit and pleased I took that route to start: a) I didn't have to think about calories on restricted days, therefore, I didn't think about food and b) because the milkshake was so restricting, choosing what to eat after the two weeks were up, has made me more aware of not to go over my calorie limit – and I don't want to.

ANITA, 51

I'd find them off-putting, but if you enjoy them or find them convenient, there's no reason why you shouldn't use them – so long as you eat a varied diet on Feast Days!

Savouring the flavour

Unless you have chosen meal replacements, one good way to make your Fast Days more enjoyable is finding ways to add flavour without adding too many calories: which means that spices, fresh herbs, and lower-calorie sauces come into their own to add depth and keep your taste buds entertained.

Take your pick from:

Chilli – flakes are brilliant for pepping up soups, stews and baked beans; one study also suggests they might help with fat-burning and increasing the metabolism. But go easy – they pack a punch. Chopped fresh chillies are delicious too but need even more caution.

Hot Chilli Sauce is another easy way to liven things up. It contains more calories than the flakes but you need very little.

Fresh herbs are great as an addition to a salad: the most versatile are chives and basil. Try chives with scrambled eggs or with other herbs in an omelette, basil torn up and added to tomato-based soups or stews/sauces. Rocket or young spinach leaves work well both as a salad crop and added to soup or stews to add body and taste.

Garlic – low in calories and a little goes a very long way. It's much less potent if you roast it along with other vegetables – break into cloves but leave them in their pink skins till they're roasted, then squeeze it out of the skins as a puree. You can even spread on a slice of bread if you're brave, it's as unctuous as butter.

Horseradish/Wasabi – I love the scary-hot tang of wasabi (the green horseradish you get in pre-packed sushi trays or in a tube) even though the tiniest quantity is eye-watering. Great to take your mind off fasting, though!

Miso – this Japanese fermented paste comes in jars or tubes and adds a meaty (though it's veggie) flavour to all sorts of dishes, and also works as a very low calorie soup stirred with boiling water in a mug. You can also buy it as powdered sachets ready to make into soup – more convenient to take to work.

Mustard – like horseradish, it's hot and tasty and works with cheese, ham and other cold meats.

Pickles/chutneys – I am addicted to all things sweet and sour, including pickles and chutneys. Be mindful of the sugar content, but a small amount, calorie-counted, can give you a hit of flavour – spread some very thinly on a slice of bread, add a slice of low-cal cheese and grill for a Fast Day cheese on toast…

Salsa – either buy fresh, in jars (still surprisingly tasty) or make your own (see the recipe under Ingredient Inspiration) – it's great as an accompaniment to fish, lean meat or Quorn/Veggie burgers and as it contains no sugar, is a much better bet than tomato ketchup.

Soy sauce – is salty but definitely adds zing, as does **Worcestershire sauce**.

Vinegars – cider or wine vinegars can work well as a dressing without oil, as can balsamic, though the latter is slightly more calorific as it's sweet, so measure it and count in your calorie allowance – it's around 16 cals per tablespoon. I also love tomatoes baked in the oven with a few drops of balsamic and then served with fresh herbs like basil or thyme.

What NOT to eat on your Fast Day

Of course, you can eat what you like – up to your calorie limit – but here are some things that many people avoid on Fast Days:

Fruit and fruit juice
Juiced and many whole fruits may upset your blood sugar balance due to the natural sugars – you could be hit by cravings by 11am which is NOT what you want. The most useful exception is fresh berries – whole strawberries, blueberries and raspberries won't give you quite the same intense sugar hit, but they are intensely flavoured. Frozen berries can also work well when fresh aren't in season – blueberries and raspberries are particularly nice.

Refined carbohydrates
White bread, potatoes and white rice are particularly likely to give you that carb high that will then make you hungry 'on the rebound'. Complex carbohydrates – seeded rolls, brown rice, sweet potatoes – will have a less dramatic effect but you won't get a very big portion of these foods if you want to stay within your Fast Day calorie limit.

One approach to helping you find the foods that won't trigger sugar spikes, is the Glycaemic Index, which measures how fast different foods are converted to sugar in the blood stream. It's not just the basic foods that vary – the variety and even the cooking method of something like potatoes has a dramatic effect. So boiled potatoes cause much less of a spike than a jacket spud.

I've added some links about GI in the Resources section. But remember, it's about finding what works for you. One 5:2 convert swears by a small jacket potato as her main meal on a Fast Day!

Alcoholic drinks
These are high in calories and won't fill you up – on an empty stomach, they could lower your willpower, too.

Confession time: I know it's nothing to be proud of, but I have been known to save 100 calories for a glass of wine if I am going to the pub. Obviously, you shouldn't be having 20% of your calories as alcohol on a regular basis but wine or particularly brut champagne/cava can be a very nice pick-me-up. Two glasses, though, and you probably won't be able to resists what everyone else is eating …

Breakfasts

For years, received diet wisdom has held that breakfast is the most important meal of the day – but I'm one of many 5:2 dieters to discover to my surprise that I don't actually need it. In fact, on Fast Days, many people seem to find that the longer they can delay their first meal, the less hungry they feel.

However, if you can't face the day without it, there are lots of options for you.

Ready-made options

With ready-made breakfast options, it makes sense to get label-savvy – so many cereals are high in sugar that they could really knock you off course.

Cereals

Many 5:2 dieters avoid sweetened packet cereals, due to the blood sugar high/low that I mentioned in the introduction to this part of the book. Also the portions when you measure them out are really tiny. Porridge or All Bran are probably a better bet, or some low-sugar mueslis including mainstream brands like Alpen – look for higher fibre and lower carbohydrate counts on the label.

Cereal bars

These are marketed as healthy alternatives to normal cereals, but have many of the same drawbacks – most come in at 100 calories or so but are so sweet you'll be craving another one within an hour or less. I used to love one particular brand – but always ended up eating two, which defeated the object, I could have had a normal biscuit instead for fewer calories! A test of cereal bars carried out by *Which?* in the UK showed that one contained almost 4 teaspoons' worth of sugar. So again, be wary.

Porridge/Oatmeal

Nutritionists often recommend oats as a good breakfast cereal because they release energy in the body slowly. For portion control, a pre-measured packet like Oatso Simple or Quaker Instant Oatmeal works well for some dieters. It's better to make it with water to save calories, but if you can't bear it, semi-skimmed milk will still keep the calories under 200.

Oatso Simple Original with water – 98 calories
Oatso Simple Original with 180mg semi-skimmed milk –
    188 calories
Quaker Instant Oatmeal, Lower Sugar Flavours – 120 calories
Quaker Oatmeal Perfect Portions Cinnamon Instant Oatmeal –
    160 calories

Out and about, Pret a Manger do a **Porridge with Compote** for 267 calories or without for 242 calories – a hefty chunk out of your allowance, but filling and easy. **Starbucks Perfect Porridge with Skimmed Milk** is 205 for a pot, as is **Sainsbury's Express Porridge Pot.**

Smoothies

Pure fruit smoothies might seem tempting for a meal on the go, but they are not ideal, for the reasons given in the previous chapter – fruit can play havoc with blood sugar and make you hungry very fast. But those with yogurt, oats and other slowly digested ingredients may be a better bet. Look at the calorie counts but also at the sugar/carbohydrate count on the label – the lower the better.

Yogurt

There are so many varieties of yogurt that you need to be label savvy. I love the richness of Greek yogurt, and prefer taking a tiny portion of that on a Fast Day to more of a low-fat variety. As always, follow your taste buds. A good breakfast option can be a natural low-fat, low-carb yogurt and then add a few nuts or seeds (again, measured carefully) to stave off hunger pangs later: sunflower or pumpkin seeds will work, along with a few fresh seasonal strawberries or frozen raspberries or blueberries.

Home-made and Home-cooked breakfasts

Something on toast …

Who can resist toast …? It's the crack cocaine of the carbohydrate world for me: one slice is never enough. So it can be a risky choice on a fast day. But if you can stick to one or two slices without butter it can make your mornings more bearable. A medium slice of Hovis Granary Wholemeal is 92 cals: a slice from one of their smaller wholemeal loaves is around 57 .

The following are for the topping only and I've used a range of different brands – most supermarkets will have similar products:

Food	Calories
Medium poached egg	75–85
Heinz Snap Pot Baked Beans 200g	144
Sunpat Crunchy Peanut Butter – 1 teaspoon (5g)	30
Philadelphia Extra Light Cream Cheese (10g)	11
Philadelphia with Cadbury Dairy Milk (10g)	30
Tesco – Sliced Honey Roast Ham	24
Asda Singles Light Cheese Slice (each)	38

Go to work on an egg?

Eggs are protein-rich, but they can also be very satisfying, especially at breakfast, so it's worth considering them. Poaching or boiling are the least calorific ways of preparing them, but they can also be fried using the oil sprays you can buy, which typically work out at 1 calorie per spray – not as tasty as butter, but they won't eat up your entire allowance either.

BASIC SCRAMBLED EGG RECIPE: 155 calories

I know most of us have our own ways of making scrambled egg, but here's one that always works:

- Take two eggs (1 large egg has approx. 70 calories), crack into a mug or cup, add 2 tablespoons (30ml : 15 calories) of semi-skimmed milk.

- Beat well with a fork till yolks and whites are combined. Season with salt and pepper.

- Spray a small non-stick saucepan with low-calorie or no-calorie spray and put on low/medium heat: the more slowly you cook them, the less rubbery they'll be.

- Add egg mixture and cook for one minute without beating. Then begin to move the mix around the pan with a spoon or spatula, until mixture begins to set or thicken, depending on how you prefer your eggs. Cook thoroughly if you are pregnant or immune-compromised. Remember mixture will keep heating as long as it's in the hot pan so serve immediately.

Additions:
- Fresh herbs, chopped
- Chilli flakes
- Mushrooms pre-fried in no-cal spray
- Chopped ham or smoked salmon – a little goes a long way

Serving suggestion: Instead of serving on toast, use no-cal spray to fry large Portobello/field mushrooms for 4–5 minutes (turning halfway) – and top with the eggs.

Anytime Omelettes

I'm a fan of omelettes because to me they seem more complete without the addition of the (calorific) toast.

BASIC OMELETTE RECIPE: 140 calories

- Break two medium/50g eggs (70 cals each) into a bowl and whisk well till combined. Season with salt and pepper.

- Use a small non-stick frying or omelette pan and no/low-cal spray and heat the pan till it's hot but not burning: apparently you should be able to touch it with the back of your hand but I would caution against doing this!

- Add the egg and keep the mix moving so that all the uncooked egg has contact with the pan – do this for 1–2 minutes.

- Then hold the pan at an angle and let the omelette move forwards towards the site of the pan – use the spatula to lift a third of the omelette back on itself. It's a folding process! Do it again for the other side until it's a cigar shape!

- Again, you can add extras, either to the centre of the omelette when it's part cooked but before the fold, or to the basic mixture.

Home-made Porridge/Oatmeal

There are many different brands available, so pick your favourite: I am a huge fan of Flahavan's Irish Porridge Oats – they are so creamy and yummy, even made with water.

Oatmeal brands have microwave or hob cooking instructions on the pack. A 40g serving of Flahavan's made with 240nl skimmed milk is 237 calories.

Home-made Bircher Muesli

This is how I like my oats. I first discovered it on holiday in the posh hotel buffet, and it's filling and healthy. It's also almost effortless and tastes a lot yummier than it sounds. The only problem is that it makes a very small portion in a bowl … but we're getting used to those doll's-house-sized portions.

BASIC BIRCHER MUESLI: 168 calories

This is a small portion but very filling…

25g porridge oats (97 cals)
25ml semi skimmed milk (12 cals) or apple juice (11 cals)
plus a teaspoon (5g) of sultanas (15 cals)

- Mix the two together, put in a bowl or plastic container in the fridge overnight, covered.

- In the morning, if it's a little bit dry, add slightly more liquid. Grate half a small apple over the top (27 cals), mix in and 2 tablespoons (30ml) of plain low-fat yogurt (17 cals) plus any of the ingredients suggested above for porridge – berries are especially good.

- Take it to work in a plastic pot!

Things to add to porridge or oatmeal

Food	Calories
Teaspoon honey	20
Teaspoon (5g) sunflower seeds	30
Teaspoon (5g) dried sultanas	15
½ grated very small apple (approx. 50g)	27
Raspberries – 20 (frozen are fine: add them to unheated oats straight from the freezer before cooking when fresh berries aren't available)	20 (1 cal each!)
Blueberries: 50 berries	39
Tablespoon (15g) low-fat yogurt	Check label!
Cadbury Bournville Cocoa powder 1 teaspoon	18
Teaspoon of powdered cinnamon (a teaspoon may be too much!)	6

Cool lunches and hot dinners

Again, I've split this into ready-made meals that I and other dieters have found filling and tasty – and then suggestions for home-made dishes. You can obviously have them for lunch, dinner – or breakfast, if you feel like it. It's your diet …

Ready-made main dishes

If you choose to eat one main meal a day, then it will be really easy to find ready meals that come in at 500-600 calories a serving. As a pointer, try to choose meals with a balance of protein and carbohydrate, to keep you from getting hungry again too quickly (a chocolate cheesecake or brownie dessert might come in under the limit but will probably drive you crazy with hunger again within a couple of hours).

If you're planning two or three meals a day, I've taken recommendations from our forum members from the main brands and supermarkets to help you choose. If you haven't tasted diet meals for a while, you may be in for a pleasant surprise!

Innocent Veg Pots – these vegetable and pulse-based dishes, which tend to be stews or casseroles based on various cuisines, including Indian, Thai and Mexican. They are filling, though the presence of lots of beans and fibre can have explosive consequences … just saying. The calorie count varies from around 215 to over 300. Many supermarkets now do very similarly packaged own brand versions.

Kirstys.co.uk – their ready meals are popular with several 5:2 regulars: these healthy versions of classic dishes come from the company featured on TV's *Dragon's Den*. They're stocked in Sainsbury's and other stores: particular forum favourites are … Moroccan Vegetables with Quinoa (276 calories) and Cottage Pie with Sweet Potato Mash (288 calories).

Marks & Spencer Simply Fuller Longer range does what it says on the packet, and the dishes are formulated to satisfy the appetite for as long as possible. They're not all low-calorie so do check the label – the fish dishes tend to be the lowest in calories e.g. King Prawns, Lochmuir Hot Smoked Salmon With Couscous & A Lemon Vinaigrette is 320 calories! The **Count on Us** range is also recommended, especially the Fish Pie (345 calories) and 295 calorie Roast Pork Loin In Gravy, New Potatoes, Savoy Cabbage & Carrots.

Waitrose's Love Life You Count range has lots of fans: they do apply the branding to a lot of different products but the You Count ones tend to offer a main meal dish at around 300 calories, like the Chicken, Wild Mushrooms and Vegetables at 318 or Beef and Red Wine Casserole at 297.

Tesco's Eat Live Enjoy range includes Chilli King Prawn Noodles (275 per pack) and the **Light Choices** Mushroom Risotto with 360.

Morrisons NuMe Range gets a really big thumbs up from the forum, with the Chilli and Potato Wedges

(313) , Spinach and Ricotta Cannelloni (292) and the Cumberland Pie (297) voted tasty and filling – though apparently you have to be quick as they fly off the shelf!

Asda Chosen by You Chicken Sizzler is a hit at 292 calories and **Sainsbury's Be Good to Yourself** range has lots of options – suggested picks are the hearty Shepherd's Pie (349 calories) and the Tomato and Basil Chicken (372).

The **Cook** stores and online shop are rated highly, too – they're frozen meals presented in a home-made way. Their latest range includes Salmon Fishcakes with Thai Seasoning at 230 calories per portion, and Paella with chicken, chorizo, peppers and peas at 307. They also do a good range of vegetarian dishes and smaller pots for lunch, and will deliver a Diet Meals Weekly Box.

Most supermarkets also make vegetable-based side dishes which come in smaller packs than the standard ready meals. They're often designed for sharing, but eating the whole pack of Cauliflower Cheese or one of the Indian side dishes can still come in at under 300 cals and often the dishes are satisfying in themselves. I like the Spinach Dhal from Waitrose – the spices in veggie side dishes mean your meal is big on flavour, but low in calories.

One tip: If you choose a diet option ready-meal, try adding your own spices or fresh herbs to add flavour – I've mixed in a little French or wholegrain mustard into a thin cauliflower cheese sauce which had no discernible cheese, or you could add just a little low-fat cream cheese to a sauce or curry side dish without adding too many calories … soy or chilli sauces are also great.

Ready-made soups

Making your own soup is easy and cheap, but for a no-hassle option, I often buy ready-made and the flavours and brands keep on improving (they used to taste very salty but I find the newer versions less heavy handed). It's a great option in colder weather when a salad, however low in calories, doesn't quite seem to fill you up. There's also scientific evidence that eating soup keeps you fuller, for longer, because it stays in the stomach for longer.

One brand that gets the thumbs up is the **Glorious Skinny** – the Azteca is spicy, with chunks of pepper and tortilla (half a pot = 90 cals), while the Fragrant Thai Carrot is very warming and 119 calories for a portion.

The Yorkshire Provender Company has some lovely dishes. Tomato and Red Pepper with Wensleydale is a little higher in calories than some (176 calories for half a pot), but the chewy pieces of cheese are delicious. Beetroot and Horseradish comes in at 168 cals for half a pot.

The original pioneers in this area, **New Covent Garden Soup**, continue to make a fantastic and wide range of soups and are very widely available. Forum members particularly like the Souper Green (90 calories per half carton) and the seasonal varieties like Winter Broth with Bacon and Kale (½ pot, 96 calories). They also make soups with portions of vegetables that are steamed in the microwave and added as part of the cooking process – the Red Thai Sweet Potato and Coconut is one of my favourites as a main meal soup, 256 calories.

Supermarket own brand soups – still in the plastic tubs which you can microwave – tend to be cheaper and still have great ingredients and taste.

I like the **Marks & Spencer** Spicy Red Lentil and Tomato which is 150 cals. for half a pot, but incredibly filling.

The **Tesco** Tomato and Basil is 'absolutely delicious', our group reports, and 210 calories for the whole pot.

Asda's range includes Broccoli and Stilton and Beef Broth – 'very tasty and low in price'.

Waitrose Love Life Chargrilled Vegetable Soup Waitrose Love Life is full of flavour and 100 calories per portion, while **Sainsbury's** Chicken and Sweetcorn is a filling 161 per half pot.

Don't rule out Cup-a-soups or tinned soups – really convenient and cheaper than the fresh varieties. For example, the **Crosse and Blackwell** Best of British Broccoli and Stilton is 'lovely and rich' and 204 calories for the whole tin – and **Baxter's** Healthy Minestrone with Wholemeal Pasta is hearty and tempting, 79 calories for half a tin.

I often eat a portion of soup for lunch and dinner – with a slice of bread or Ryvita to add some crunch (I noticed when I tried to eat only soup, I missed the texture of other foods as much as the calories). Again, I like the convenience of having my day's meals in a single pot – great for work.

Ready-made grains and noodles

Pasta won't offer you much bulk for your calories, but if you want something more solid than soup, and as convenient, you could look at the microwaveable rice pouches which have extra flavours and spicing built in – one of these will probably add up to around 400 cals for the packet, so serve in two portions, perhaps with some frozen veg added: I'd definitely gravitate towards the brown rice versions as white rice will usually make you hungry again, much faster.

Tilda Roasted Pepper and Courgette Steamed Brown Basmati Rice contains 176 calories for half a pack, or the Veetee Vegetable Biryani is 174 for half a pack.

We're moving towards Home-Made in this category but there's been a lot of talk on diet forums lately about 'no calorie' shirataki noodles which are made of a kind of yam and are supposed to leave you full but not add to your calorie count. They're so popular they've been sold out wherever I go but I've heard mixed reports. Yes, they're filling, and they can work well combined with a stir fry or some prawns or lean meat. However, don't expect them to taste too much like 'real' noodles. They can also have a slightly fishy smell. Shirataki noodles are also available with tofu as part of the mix which may make them more satisfying. You can buy them online or via health food or Asian speciality shops.

Preparing couscous could count as borderline cooking, but there are various flavoured couscous brands that you put in a bowl and add boiling water to – in the UK, the Ainsley Harriott packets contain two portions of around 170–190 each – again, you can bulk them out with frozen peas or corn, or serve with a veggie sausage or burger.

Home-made and Home-cooked main meals

All the egg dishes and 'on toast' dishes from the Breakfast Section will work equally well at another time of day: beans on toast is one of those dishes you can eat without anyone really noticing you're on a diet – especially nice if you add some chilli flakes or sauce!

The best site I've found to allow you to select favourite ingredients, cooking time and calorie counts is the BBC Good Food site, bbcgoodfood.com – there's a specific section with recommended 200–400 calorie dishes including Healthy Fish and Chips, and Full English Frittata. You can also save all your favourites into your own recipe binder if you register, and read other reviews of each recipe posted by users.

In this section, I'll stick to simple dishes which barely count as 'recipes' – they're more suggestions for fast and easy meals when you don't want to spend too much time cooking or in reach of temptations.

Meat and two veg

You obviously need to be a little more careful about your meat and two veg meals while you're fasting, but it certainly doesn't mean giving them up!

Over the page, I've created a mix and match table with some suggestions for combinations and portion size: treat all the calorie counts as a guideline and double check on the back of your packs. Most steamed/boiled green veg come in at around 30–35 calories per 100 grams though peas and corn are higher in calories.

Meat/Fish	Veg 1	Veg 2	Total cals:
Salmon Portion size: small steak, 100g, 135 calories	**Mangetout/snow peas** 100g 32 calories	**Mushrooms** fried in no-cal spray 60g 10 calories	177
Tuna Portion size: 1 steak, 75g, 115 calories	**Sweet corn** 75g canned 50 cals	**Spinach** ½ cup cooked & drained 32 cals	197
Prawns Portion size: 100g, 80 calories	**Roast tomatoes** 10 cherry tomatoes 30 cals, roasted with no cal spray & 5ml balsamic 5 cals	**Green beans** 100g approx. 30 cals	145
Chicken Portion size: 100g breast fillet, 100–140 calories	**Broccoli** 1 cup, steamed 30 cals	**Sliced mixed peppers** 80g 25 cals	155– 195
Turkey Portion size: 100g breast fillet, 100–140 calories	**Baby Carrots** Frozen handful 80g 18 cals	**Cauliflower** 100g steamed 25 cals	143– 183
Quorn burger/ banger Portion size: Burger 50g, 80 calories banger x 1 50–60 calories	**Sweet potato** small: 133g 105 calories	**Garden peas** 50g 34 cals	189– 219

One pot meals

The recipes that follow are simple and fresh and infinitely adaptable: use them as the basis for healthy, nutritious and low-calorie meals on Fast Days.

EASY VEGETABLE CURRY: 150 calories per portion (makes two portions)

Replace the veg with any others in season – adjusting the calories, of course. Also, you can serve with a portion of meat or fish as listed in the previous section.

1 tsp (5ml) oil	200g cauliflower or
2 cloves garlic, crushed	broccoli, broken into
1 onion, finely chopped	small florets
1 tsp chilli powder	100g carrots, sliced
1 tsp ground ginger	100g potatoes, diced
1 tsp turmeric powder	1 tsp tomato puree
100g green beans, sliced	20g sultanas

- Cook the garlic and onion in the oil in a large pan for five minutes, before adding the spices and cooking gently for a further minute.

- Add all the vegetables and 300ml of water, then add the other ingredients.

- Heat till water boils, then reduce the heat and cover – it'll be ready in half an hour.

This keeps well in the fridge for 48 hours if you want to save till your next Fast Day.

MEDITERRANEAN ROAST VEG: 148 calories per portion
(makes four portions)

This is good with whatever herbs or spices you fancy – try chilli flakes. Mushrooms, baby corn or slices of butternut squash (in 1 cm slices so they bake through) taste great too.

    3 tbsp. olive oil
    4 large courgettes sliced
    5 plum tomatoes sliced
    2 aubergines sliced
    1 large garlic bulb (don't peel)
    A bunch of rosemary, broken into sprigs, or oregano, or thyme

- Heat oven to 220°C/200°C fan/gas 7. Drizzle a third of the oil into a tin or ovenproof dish then layer the vegetables across the dish – with the garlic head in the middle. Poke the herbs in amongst the layered veg, add 1 tablespoon of olive oil over the top and season.

- Roast for 45 minutes – 1 hour until the vegetables are charred around the edges, adding remaining oil during cooking. You can use less but it's virtuous already!

- Serve with the still-wrapped cloves of garlic, to be squeezed out over the vegetables.

If you make more than you need, make soup: add to a large saucepan with water and a tin of tomatoes, bring to the boil. Adjust the water to make the consistency you like. When it's cooled down, blend in pan with a stick blender.

SO EASY STIR FRY: 160 calories per portion
(makes two very generous portions)

Another base recipe that you can adapt with different veg –
peppers and spring onion/scallion would be nice. Or buy stir-
fry veg packs from supermarkets/convenience stores.

If you want to use meat or fish, pre-fry these in the oil to
make sure they're cooked through. Then set aside, fry veg in
the same pan and heat through all the ingredients after adding
soy and chilli sauce.

Alternatively, add thinly sliced tofu at the same time as the
vegetables, or a beaten egg, just after the soy and chilli sauce
stage for veggie protein options.

1 tbsp vegetable oil
1 red chilli, sliced (leave out if you don't like hot food)
1 garlic clove, sliced
500g mixed vegetables such as pak choi, baby corn and
    broccoli
1½ tbsp soy sauce
2 tbsp sweet chilli sauce

- Heat the oil in a wok or frying pan, then fry the chilli and garlic for one min.

- Add the vegetables and make sure they've all been coated in all. Fry for
  2–3 mins.

- Add the soy and chilli sauce then cook for a further 2–3 mins until the veg
  are tender.

Soups

SPICY INDIAN LENTIL & TOMATO: 130 calories per portion
(makes two portions)

A very simple, warming soup made from the things you have in your larder. Double up the portions and freeze if you like.

1 chopped onion
Pinch of chilli flakes
2 tbsp of red lentils
1 400g tin chopped tomatoes
500ml vegetable stock (I used Marigold bouillon)
Coriander leaf, to taste (maybe ½ bunch)

- Put all the ingredients, except the coriander, in a pan together and heat till simmering.

- Cover and cook for twenty minutes till the lentils are soft.

- Add the coriander, cook for one minute and blend with stick blender. Season and serve.

MUSHROOM TOM YUM SOUP: 40 calories per portion
(makes four portions)

Very tasty, very fast and very low in calories.

  1 litre chicken or vegetable stock

  1–2 tbsp tom yum paste

  200g fresh mushrooms (ideally a mixture including oyster
    and shiitake)

  4 dried shiitake mushrooms rehydrated in water (remove
    hard edges)

  Juice of 1 lime

  Fish sauce to taste – around 1 tablespoon

  1 sliced red chilli

  Coriander leaf to taste

- Bring the stock to the boil in a large pan, add the paste and then the
  mushrooms.

- Simmer for five minutes before adding the other ingredients. Season and
  add more fish sauce if required before serving.

GREEN AND WHITE SUPER SOUP: 76 calories per portion
(makes two portions)

Super-vitamins, super-easy.

½ bunch spring onions, chopped
1 tsp oil
1 small potato, peeled and diced
500ml vegetable stock (made with 5g Marigold bouillon)
140g bag watercress, spinach and rocket

- Cook the spring onions/scallions in olive oil until soft: add the potato and cook for two more minutes.

- Add stock and simmer till potato is tender (10–15 minutes depending on size of the dice).

- Add the bag of salad, simmer for a minute then use stick blender to blend till smooth. Season and serve.

ALMOST INSTANT CORN CHOWDER: 115 calories per portion
(one portion)

This is a really comforting and simple store-cupboard soup – with a chilli kick.

1 medium spring onion/scallion
300ml stock made with 2.5g/½ teaspoon Marigold Swiss
    Vegetable Bouillon
100g frozen sweet corn
Pinch chilli flakes
20ml fresh semi-skimmed/2% fat milk

- Use no-cal spray to fry the onion for 2 minutes
- Add all the ingredients except the milk, simmer for five minutes, then add milk and blend lightly with stick blender. Season & serve.

Stuffed vegetables

Vegetables make ideal 'carriers' for ingredients – low in calories but colourful and tasty for Fast Days!

Portabello/breakfast mushrooms are large and flat, as big as beef burgers, and make brilliant containers for fillings. I tend to grill or microwave them with the fillings – they're so low in calories that you could also serve them as 'burgers' if they've been grilled or fried in no-cal spray, in a bun!

PHILLY MUSHROOMS: 66 calories for two

- Take 2 large flat mushrooms (approx. 125g: 20 calories) and wipe with kitchen towel. Spoon 30g (2tbsp) Philadelphia Light with Herbs or Chives into the mushrooms and top with chopped herbs or black pepper: either grill for 2 minutes until hot through or microwave for 30–45 seconds.

- The Mediterranean filling for the avocado recipe below also works well in mushrooms or peppers.

STUFFED AVOCADO: 125 calories plus your choice of filling

Avocados are high in fat but filling and tasty – you can serve them cold, of course, but also hot if you want to try something different. Their shape makes a nice 'bowl' for all sorts of fillings. Use half a medium Hass avocado (125 calories): save the other half in the fridge to use later the same day – store with the stone still inside and a little lemon juice on the cut surface to stop it discolouring. Add whatever fillings you fancy:

- Guacamole style: add shop-bought salsa, or a mix of two cherry chopped tomatoes, sprinkling of chilli flakes, and half a chopped medium spring onion (less than 10 calories)
- Cream cheese style: add 1 tablespoon of Philadelphia light (any flavour, 20 calories) – this can be microwaved for approx. 20–30 seconds or grilled for approx. 5 minutes to serve as a kind of pate with Ryvita or other crackers: spray first with 0-cal cooking spray before grilling.

- Rocket and balsamic vinegar: pour 1tbsp (15ml: 15 cals) vinegar into the hollow of the avocado, add a good handful of rocket leaves (20g is loads and just 4 cals) and grind plenty of pepper and sea salt on top.
- Prawns and lime: 60g of cooked prawns (approx. 45 cals) plus half a lime (under 10 cals for the juice) to serve. Or use low-cal dressing of your choice.
- Mediterranean Hot: spray the avocado with no-cal cooking spray and grill for five minutes or microwave for 20–30 seconds. In the hollow, place a mix of 1 chopped sun-dried tomato with oil drained off, two stoned olives, a few capers, ½ spring onion/scallion, some torn basil or rocket leaves (filling is less than 20 calories).

QUICKEST EVER STUFFED PEPPER: 92 calories for two halves

- Halve a medium red or yellow pepper (31 cals) and pull out seeds/ white core. Add three cherry tomatoes to each half (18 cals for 6) and medium spring onion/scallion (5 cals), cut into small slices with a knife or scissors. Top with 30g Philadelphia Light (any savoury flavour, 40 cals) plus other flavourings from suggested in the Tips section.

- Grill for approx. 10–12 minutes or roast in oven 200°C for around 30 minutes, till the pepper flesh is soft and the edges are charred.

Salads

A pre-washed bag of salad contains very few calories – and is a canvas for a great Fast Day salad. Make your own salad by adding any of these ingredients.

Salad Ingredient	Calories
½ bag pre-washed salad – whichever you like! – see label	15–30
Cherry tomatoes – per tomato	3
Sliced red or green pepper – per pepper	30
Beetroot, 50g cooked	16
Sweet corn – 50g drained from tin	40–50
Spring onion – Medium	8
Parmesan – shaved thinly with potato slicer – 10g shavings	40
Cottage cheese: varies depending on fat content – per 100g	60–100
Wafer thin ham (deli style) – slice varies – per slice	10–15
Wafer thin turkey (deli style) – slice varies – per slice	8–15
Cooked prawns – 50g	40
Smoked salmon – 1 60g slice	80–100

Artichoke hearts: depends on size of can – per portion	25-50
Pumpkin seeds: teaspoon (5g)	29
Pine nuts: teaspoon (5g)	35
Sunflower seeds: teaspoon (5g)	30
Buffalo mozzarella, ½ container (2.2 oz/60g.)	170
Chopped apple: ½ small apple (approx. 50g)	27
Walnuts: teaspoon (5g)	34
Whole boiled egg	70–80

A–Z Ingredient Inspiration

This section is designed to give you a little boost if you're bored and are looking for quick, new ideas.

Food	Ideas	Calories
A is for Asparagus	Super nutritious and filling, and delicious, either steamed, boiled or — easiest of all — microwaved. Serve with sea salt and pepper, lemon juice, or a nice poached egg on the side to dip into! You can also pre-cook and then grill. It's a great summer dish.	5 spears = 25
A is also for Almonds	These are so good and although like all nuts they're calorific, a small handful can be very filling. I've also used them ground — a teaspoon mixed with yogurt and berries, gives you a hint of sweetness while containing negligible carbs, so you'll stave off the hunger pangs for longer.	1 whole = 7 1 Teaspoon = (5g) 31
B is for Beetroot	You might have gathered that I am a bit of a beetroot fiend, especially the sort that's been flavoured with chilli, or baked with cumin powder and served with a little low-fat yogurt or cumin. It's very good for you, and makes a delicious salad with rocket, cherry tomatoes, balsamic vinegar and some chopped fresh apple. I also like it with fresh mozzarella — the kind that comes floating in water.	50g cooked = 16

B is also for Broccoli	Another super-food. Horrible over-cooked, but steaming works well, or have you tried frying till it almost goes black? The edges caramelise if you slice through the florets into 3mm/¼ inch slices, then heat some spray oil in a pan till very hot, and fry on both sides. You need the extractor fan for this one or an open window as it can smoke but it's great with pepper and sea salt, soy sauce or chilli sauce, and very low in calories.	100g = 38
C is for Chocolate	Yum. Etc. You can't have too much of it, but two or four squares of the dark, expensive kind can be enough to satisfy a craving. It's sweet, but not too sweet, and high in anti-oxidants, too.	10g (4 small squares) = 58
D is for Dijon mustard	Or any kind of mustard. I add it to lots of savoury dishes to give a low-calorie kick — there are calories in it but it's so hot that you only need a little.	1 teaspoon (5ml) = 15
E is for Edamame beans	Those whole pods that are served in Asian restaurants are available frozen to eat at home, and they're filling, nutritious and can satisfy a snack craving.	50g = 61
F is for low-fat Feta cheese	This has a strong, salty taste, so a little goes a long way. Try in a Greek salad with lots of tomato, black olives and cucumber, perhaps with some red wine vinegar or a ready-made lower calorie dressing.	50g = 100–120

G is for Ginger	One of your best friends for extra flavour during Fast Days. I am a big fan of the clean taste of pickled ginger that's served with sushi – I'm addicted to it on its own!	25g (plenty!) = 10–15
H is for Ham	Great for when you're having a savoury craving. Parma is the expensive sort, try 2 slices with 6 thin slices of melon.	For melon and ham = 80
I is for Ices	They don't have to be out of bounds if you choose carefully. A Solero is the dieter's friend on hot days or look for Italian style ice-cream (typically less fatty than American style) or a creamy low-fat frozen yogurt (check the calories though as some can be higher than normal ice-cream).	Solero = 90 1 2.5 oz. Calories vary for Italian style and for frozen yogurt
J is for Jelly	Sugar-free jellies can help overcome a sweet craving with negligible calories.	3–10
K is for Kiwi Fruits	Often overlooked – maybe because of their unpromising exterior. But inside there's a frenzy of vitamin C. They're also helpful if you suffer from poor sleeping patterns – try one or two an hour before bed!	46
L is for Lentils	Cheap red lentils make a great basis for soup – see the recipe – and the 'gourmet' Puy variety are extremely filling and provide a nutritious and tasty base for a salad.	100g ready to eat Puy lentils = 130

M is for Marmite	Love it or hate it, we all know that a little of this yeasty spread goes a long way. Great on crisp breads or a single slice of toast. I also like Marmite flavoured cheese bites too: 85 calories for a portion.	4g = 10
N is for Noodles	Try the Shirataki 'no calorie' noodles which can be found in the chiller section and contain fewer than 20 cals (sometimes none at all) per serving. The ones with tofu taste less 'fishy' and it's best to use a strong flavoured sauce and also to 'dry roast' them for a minute in a hot pan before using!	Less than 20 cals per serving
O is for Oreo Cookies	Maybe it's because they look so cute but I adore Oreos – and the mini biscuits can give you a sweet hit without too many calories if you can stop at one or two	1 cookie = 52 ½ pack of mini cookies = 60
P is for Popsicles	Make your own low-cal popsicles or ice pops with sugar-free squash, diluted fruit juice, low-fat yogurt or pureed fruit. Use a reusable mould and go wild!	Depends on what you add
Q is for Quinoa	Quinoa – which those in the know pronounce 'keen-wa' is a seed originally grown by the Incas which is used as a grain in pilaffs or as a stuffing. It's very high protein so a little will fill you up and you can use it in salads or other dishes that are normally made with rice.	100g cooked = 100–110
R is for Ricotta	A lovely light Italian cheese with a mousse-like texture for dips, sauces or even as a substitute for mayonnaise in salads which need 'binding.' Check labels to get lower calorie versions.	25g = between 30–50 calories depending on brand

S is for Salsa	The shop-bought stuff can be really good but nothing beats home-made: this one improves after a day in the fridge. 1 tomato, finely diced 1 medium red pepper ½ cucumber, & ½ celery stick, finely diced 1 medium onion, chopped finely 2 tablespoons vinegar 2 tablespoons salt Pinch each chilli flakes, black pepper, oregano 1 teaspoon Worcestershire sauce Soak the onions in the vinegar and 1 tablespoon of salt. Leave overnight. Roast the pepper till the skin is charred, discard seeds and white parts, chop and add to the other chopped vegetables and onions. Add flavourings. Makes 8 portions.	14 per portion
T is for Tangerines	Easy to peel and the perfect portion size. Tangerines are also one of the newest super-foods, with re-search suggesting a chemical in the fruit can reduce the risk of heart attacks, diabetes and stroke, as well as staving off obesity.	1 small tangerine = 37
U is for Ugli fruit	I've never had one. Apparently it's a bit like a grapefruit.	½ fruit = 45

V is for Vinegar	Vinegar is under-rated. I'm not talking about the malty sort we have on chips — so unlikely to feature in a Fast Day. But the world of vinegar includes fruit vinegars, sherry, cider, red and white wine and even champagne: these are virtually calorie free. As a dressing the milder ones can work on their own, without oil, and balsamic — which does contain more calories — is fab on cooked veg as well as salad. Sweet and sour, yummy! Plus apparently it has lots of medicinal benefits including positive effects on blood pressure, cholesterol and diabetes/insulin sensitivity.	1 teaspoon balsamic = 12–16 1 teaspoon white wine vinegar = 1!
W is for Watercress	Another one of those ingredients often quoted as a super-food because of its high levels of Vitamin C and other nutrients — it was recommended in the 16th century as a treatment for scurvy. It makes a nutritious salad or soup ingredient, and scientists are investigating cancer-fighting properties, too.	100g = 11
X is for Xmas	Treats like mince pies and Christmas pud won't help with Fasts. But this diet is ideal for any kind of celebration — you can feel virtuous by simply fasting two days over the festive period, which might be a relief after so much rich food. Remember, this is for life, not just for Christmas.	
Y is for Yogurt	Remember the thin, unpleasant smelling diet yogurts of the eighties and nineties? Now you can get very palatable pots in a huge range of flavours.	Varies a great deal according to brand and fat content.

Treats, snacks and eating out

To snack or not to snack

The debate about 'grazing' or snacking is one I've touched on in the book, and generally many 5:2 Dieters do avoid eating between meals on Fast Days. But there are times when you just fancy something NOW and then it makes sense to go for the lower-calorie options rather than choose something that will undo the good you've done by fasting …

Health food shops are a good source of nuts or trail mix, but do check the nutritional values. My favourite snack food ever – Thai Chilli Rice Crackers – look as though they should be super-healthy but most are very high calorie …

Graze.com which delivers snacks in a letter-box sized container, with four mini-packs of sweet and savoury snacks including nuts, dried fruit and even chocolate mixes. Some are healthier than others but you can ask for a Light option and they usually offer the first boxes at half-price.

I tend to find I crave either something sweet or savoury, so here are some options for those moments when a mug of green tea won't do.

Savoury Snacks and Treats

Snack	Calories
Miso soup: most sachets of miso soup with tofu or sea vegetables	25–35
Air popped popcorn, 1 cup	31
Olives: 10 pitted green olives	42
Oatcake Plus 2 teaspoons (10g) Philadelphia Light Or 1 teaspoon (5g) Peanut Butter as a topping	35–50 15 30
Red Mini Babybel Light Babybel	61 40
10 almonds (1 almond is 7 calories – will fill you up for ages)	70
1 rasher of grilled bacon and a dollop of ketchup	87
17g pack of Quavers	88
Pack savoury Snack a Jacks	92–108
1 bag of ready salted French Fries (crisps)	97
25g bag of Twiglets	98
10 Pringles	100

Sweet Snacks and Treats

Snack	Calories
Sugar-free jellies	5–15
Options Hot Chocolates Belgian chocolate	40
Milky Way Mini	40
Jaffa Cake	46
Small scoop of soft-scoop vanilla ice-cream	50–60
10g 85% dark chocolate	55
2 medium peaches	76
20 cherries	80
1 McVitie's chocolate digestive	84
Thin slice of malt loaf	85
1 small banana	90
2 ginger biscuits	90
Solero ice-cream (Berry and Tropical flavours)	90
5 dried apricots	95
4 dates	96
2 Cadbury's Roses	100
1 meringue nest with 6 strawberries	100

Eating out

I am veering into the department of the obvious here but I try *not* to eat out on Fast Days as it's really hard to make good choices, plus you have no real idea how many calories you're consuming. You will have read earlier on in my diary about my Temptation Incident, where I went out planning to have soup at my favourite cafe, only to find it's not served at weekends. So I plumped for Eggs Florentine, which probably contained my entire daily allowance, but kept me full all day.

If you are out and about, make the choices you'd make for other diets – ask for bread to be taken off the table, or give it to your dining companion. Choose soups, ideally vegetable-based and non-creamy, and salads, and ask for the dressing on the side. Lean fish or chicken with veggies is not exciting but will usually give you some control. If all else fails – if you want to give into temptation or suddenly have something to celebrate – then it's even simpler. Fast tomorrow instead!

Fast Day meal plans for all tastes

You've got all the tools you need to plan your own Fast Days – but as an extra aid, I've outlined some daily meal plans, using these recipes and ready-made meals. Use them as the basis for your own meal planning if you find it useful … or go your own way! There's also a blank template for your own use.

Of course, men get an extra 100 calories on top of the 500 allowed for women – so I've added an extra Man's Ration to those days!

An asterisk after the dish means the recipe is featured in this book.

The big salad lunch day

This is one of my real meal days – a massive, delicious, no-holds-barred salad eaten outdoors with friends on a picnic. Slightly over in terms of calories, but plenty of protein and fat that kept me from getting hungry until next day.

Meal	Food	Calories
Breakfast		
Lunch	Garofalo – Bufala Mozzarella, 0.5 container (2.2 oz/60g)	174
	Peppery Baby leaf Rocket Salad, 15g	3
	Sweet fire Beetroot, 75g	30
	Balsamic Vinegar of Modena, 5ml	5
	Avocados – Raw, 49g	78
	Wholemeal mini roll	86
	Marks and Spencer – Traditional Coleslaw, 40g	132
Dinner		
Snacks		
Total		508

Optional Man Ration: 125ml of Chenin Blanc white wine (perfect with this picnic salad) = 110 calories

A soupy day on the go

A day to prove you have two fairly filling meals and a snack – or two snacks if you're male!

Meal	Food	Calories
Breakfast	Black coffee	
Lunch	Leek and Potato soup with	120
	White bread croutons	79
Dinner	Home-Made Green & White Super Soup*	76
	Chicken breast 100g	100
	Salsa	14
	Broccoli, 100g, steamed	32
	60g mushrooms fried with no-cal oil spray then heated with	10
	20g Philadelphia with Chives	32
Snacks	1 sugar-free Raspberry jelly	10
Total		473

Optional Man Ration: 1 medium banana (90 cals) or small bag of Twiglets (98 cals)

Family friendly Feast

For those days when you don't want to cook separate dishes for the family – or when you don't want anyone to notice you're on a diet. Simply eat the same dishes but serve extras (granola and lots of yogurt for breakfast, extra toast with butter and cheese for lunch, portion of pilau rice and chicken or prawns for dinner) to your family and they won't even notice …

Meal	Food	Calories
Breakfast	Fresh raspberries 20 25g Greek style yogurt	20 34
Lunch	Toast (1 slice) Beans (200g)	92 144
Dinner	Mushroom Tom Yum Soup* Vegetable curry*	40 150
Snacks		
Total		480

Optional Man Ration: ⅓rd portion of Tilda microwaved wholegrain pilau = 98 calories

The big breakfast

Enjoy a super-satisfying breakfast/brunch to keep you full all day!

Meal	Food	Calories
Breakfast	2 rashers lean unsmoked back bacon	106
	2 portobello mushrooms grilled with	45
	1 tsp olive oil	40
	8 cherry tomatoes on the vine	24
	1 slice granary bread	90
	1 free range pork sausage, 86% pork, grilled	122
	1 free range egg, poached	75
Lunch		
Dinner		
Snacks		
Total		502

Optional Man Ration: 125ml freshly squeezed orange juice (63 cals), 100 grams mixed frozen berries (30 cals) – either whole, or blended together as a smoothie.

Celebration Time

If you plan it carefully, you can still go to the ball ... of course, when you're eating out, calories are approximate but these are all safe bets!

Meal	Food	Calories
Breakfast		
Lunch	1 portion Spicy Indian Lentil & Tomato soup*	130
Dinner	7 cherry tomatoes,	21
	7 carrot sticks	35
	4 cucumber sticks	4
	2 tablespoons hummus	23
	2 tablespoons salsa	15
	1 grilled chicken wing	55
	2 pieces nigri salmon sushi	125
Snacks	Cava, 125 ml/4.2 fl. oz.	94
Total		502

Optional Man Ration: 2 x Grissini Italian breadsticks (40 cals), 1 tablespoon guacamole (25), 1 mini cocktail sausage (30) = 95

Blank Planning Template

Use to plan and then monitor your own Fast Days. Record your mood and thoughts as you progress – to help you work out what's the best balance for you.

There's a downloadable, printable version via my website, kate-harrison.com/5-2diet

Date:			
Meal	**Food**	**Calories**	**Mood & comments**
Breakfast			
Lunch			
Dinner			
Snacks & drinks			
	Total		

Date:			
Meal	**Food**	**Calories**	**Mood & comments**
Breakfast			
Lunch			
Dinner			
Snacks & drinks			
	Total		

Resources, links and the last instalment of Kate's 5:2 diary

FURTHER READING,
A GLOSSARY
AND FINAL WORDS
OF ENCOURAGEMENT!

The links and resources here have been organised chapter by chapter, to help you discover more on the subjects that matter to you. Where a link is very long, I've used a 'bitly' link which is simply a way of shortening the address – just type the short link into your browser.

I've put together a free downloadable list of all the links, to make it easier to follow up internet resources directly from your computer. It's available at www.the5-2dietbook.com and will save you a lot of typing! Please do bear in mind that although I've checked through these links, I can't be responsible for any outside content.

PART ONE
THE 5:2 REVOLUTION

CHAPTER TWO:
The maths of weight loss – and why Fasting adds up

Dr John Briffa on why BMI is not the best predictor of future health: http://bit.ly/W3i2Nr

The Telegraph on the height/weight ratio as a measure of CVD risk: http://bit.ly/UYneDE

Plus summary of one study: http://1.usa.gov/SwIwLe

Abstract of study on intermittent calorie restriction by Krista Varady 1.usa.gov/fLnc4v

The Mark's Daily Apple website has a focus on 'primal living' but there's a terrific amount of information on fasting, including summaries on the science http://bit.ly/Uui9DP

CHAPTER THREE:
The Fasting Recharge

Simple description of apoptosis http://en.wikipedia.org/wiki/Apoptosis & autophagy http://en.wikipedia.org/wiki/Autophagy

Summary of various studies focusing on fighting ageing in mice http://bit.ly/SwOFHh

News article on experiment on mice genetically engineered to produce more FGF21 http://bit.ly/V8DiDM

Plastic surgeon James Johnson carried out research on people with asthma undertaking his UpDayDownDay Diet http://bit.ly/TUPKXF

Overview of fasting research by Krista Varady and Marc Hellerstein. Their review of studies was published in 2007 so is a little out of date, but contains a great summary of the diverse research: http://bit.ly/113ykL3

A more recent review http://bit.ly/ShaV4h examines more studies.

The Genesis Breast Cancer Prevention Centre in Manchester is at genesisuk.org and has run a number of studies: there's a summary of one here http://1.usa.gov/XxFkNn or download a guide to the work being done by Genesis http://bit.ly/100sv2n

These two blogs explore whether women's physiological responses to fasting are different to men's, http://bit.ly/XxFowH and http://bit.ly/X7mTNi

CHAPTER FOUR:
The Hunger Game – Fasting is Good for the Brain

Link about BDNF, a protein with a key role in brain health http://en.wikipedia.org/wiki/Brain-derived_neurotrophic_factor

Interesting pieces on the research into not only for Alzheimer's and other forms of dementia, but also strokes) http://bit.ly/V5ewTv

Fasting advocate Mark Sisson on brain function and fasting. http://bit.ly/QPanph

PART TWO:
5:2 YOUR WAY

STEP ONE:
How much do you want to lose, and how much can you afford to eat?

Myfitnesspal.com/tools

The difference between 'calories' and kilocalories.
en.wikipedia.org/wiki/Calorie

STEP TWO:
Your First Fast

Article on one recent survey about secretive male dieters.
http://bit.ly/Yu9OmL

Potassium, magnesium or calcium to reduce cramps.
http://bit.ly/TsrDvY

Kiwi fruits and sleep disorders: http://1.usa.gov/W3jwqN

The Diabetes UK site has very clear information about GI values and diets as well as lots about the disease itself.
http://bit.ly/Tv2B2Y

Science Daily has lots of interesting articles, written in fairly jargon-free language: start with this one http://bit.ly/QPeAsS then follow the links to other pieces that reflect your own interests!

STEP THREE:
Review, Revise, Revitalise

The getsomeheadspace.com site offers a free introductory trial of meditations, as well as some really useful downloads, including one on mindful eating. Read more about mindfulness & food in *The Independent* http://ind.pn/QsEwJp and *The New York Times* http://nyti.ms/U4Fis5

NHS analysis of study on exercising after fasting http://bit.ly/Vgv6Uh

PART THREE:
EATING THE 5:2 WAY

OVERVIEW

Conversion chart for metric measurements to imperial
http://bit.ly/U6n2hV

Conversions from grams to US Cups http://bit.ly/U4Ft6A

FOOD AND FASTING TIPS

How chillis might help with fat-burning and increasing the
metabolism http://bit.ly/11jyZHs

BREAKFASTS

Guide to analysing GI and other health aspects of your daily
cereal here. http://bit.ly/QPcolf

A study on the potential drawbacks of cereal bars
http://bbc.in/U4FCXC

Read about the nutritional values of different types of yogurt
http://bit.ly/V5hF5u_

MAIN MEALS

Scientific study on the satiating effect of soup
http://bbc.in/YahY4T

There's lots of Information about shirataki noodles here.
http://bit.ly/V5iFGS

Tangerines and the potential of nobiletin http://bit.ly/WFklpb

Medicinal benefits of vinegar http://bit.ly/Ssvdcg

GENERAL FASTING AND HEALTHY EATING LINKS:

The 'Horizon' Eat, Fast, Live Longer programme which inspired so many has its own page at http://www.bbc.co.uk/programmes/b01lxyzc: it no longer shows the entire programme, but there are some clips.

There's also an article by presenter Dr Mosley about his experiences on the BBC site http://bbc.in/UuhPVU as well as a similar one in the Daily Telegraph. http://bit.ly/11jCMol

RECIPES

The *Daily Telegraph* feature above also had some tasty recipe suggestions. http://bit.ly/V637jU

The excellent BBC Good Food recipes site allows you to specify courses, ingredients, preparation time and calorie counts – the user ratings are incredibly useful to. http://bit.ly/SsvbkI

Some brilliant bloggers are now posting images of their own recipes for **5:2** days: be inspired by lovely pictures and ideas. http://bit.ly/13LBfIE

FORUMS

Our 5:2 Diet Group on Facebook is very friendly, and anyone can see the entries: http://www.facebook.com/groups/the52diet but to post, you'll have to ask to join. There is also a new forum at the 5-2dietbook.com

The Mumsnet forum on 5:2 has become a treasure trove of brilliant advice and experiences – you definitely don't have to be a Mum to call on all that wisdom http://bit.ly/Tv3xUV and The Money Saving Expert Forum is less active but still useful http://bit.ly/ToawLX

Further Reading

***The Hairy Dieters: How to Love Food and Lose Weight* by the Hairy Bikers**
This recipe book gets the thumbs up from many forum members who love the Bikers' brilliant ideas for Fast Days.

***The Fast Diet: The secret of intermittent fasting* by Michael Mosley and Mimi Spencer**
Dr Mosley was the presenter of the 'Horizon' programme and his scientific background makes the science impeccable, while his co-author is strong on the practical side.

***The 2-Day Diet: Diet Two Days a Week. Eat Normally for Five* by Michelle Harvie and Tony Howell**
This book hasn't been published at the time of writing but it comes from the Genesis team in Manchester, whose work on breast cancer prevention is making a major contribution in the field, and I'm looking forward to reading it.

***The Alternate-Day Diet* by James B. Johnson and Donald R. Laub**

Johnson's book goes into a lot of detail about the science, if you want to know more. I'm not as keen on the meal plans or use of diet replacement meals, but you might be!

Glossary

5:2, 6:1, 4:3   Different variations on fasting/calorie restriction – the second number is usually the number of days you follow restrictions in your diet.

ADF   Alternate Daily Fasting – cutting down or eating nothing every other day.

Bit.ly   Nothing to do with fasting, but a very useful way of shortening long web links – you can type these directly into your browser to find a recommended web page.

BMI   Body Mass Index – simple height/weight calculation used to gauge whether someone's weight may be putting their health at risk.

BMR   Basal Metabolic Rate – i.e. what your body needs in calorie terms for basic survival, without any activity other than basic functions

DCR   Daily Calorie Requirement – also known
                 as Daily Calorie Need – an estimate of the
                 number of calories you need that factors in
                 your activity levels as well as age, height and
                 weight.

Fast Day   Fast usually means eating nothing (and, in
                 some religions, not drinking anything either).
                 However, 5:2 dieters often use it as shorthand
                 for days when they eat limited amounts.

Feast Day   Days when you eat normally. Also known as
                 Feed Days.

Kate's 5:2 Diary Part Five:

JANUARY 2013 AND BEYOND...

The way to live - for ever?

Mood: hopeful, expectant, optimistic

Weight 16 January 2013: 141 pounds

Total lost: 20 pounds

BMI: 24.2

Days on Diet: 160

My number one goal on January 1 2012 was to get back to a healthy weight, but it was a resolution I'd failed to achieve for *years*.

And now I have done it.

I know for certain it wouldn't have happened without 5:2 and I couldn't be more thrilled.

Christmas: the goose got fat, but I didn't!

Before Christmas, I was a bit nervous about how to maintain fasting with lots of social events revolving around food. I decided to be flexible, but to give up trying to fast during the holiday week between Christmas and New Year. I knew I might put a little weight on, but knew it would be temporary –

and so it's proved. My weight loss is continuing into January and most group members are reporting they've put very little weight on – or none at all – and are as enthusiastic as ever.

Winter whirlwind

It's been a whirlwind winter in other ways.

I finished the first edition of this book in November and it went on sale on Kindle at the end of the month. Within days, it was topping the diet chart, and I've had so many emails and new forum members who are every bit as excited as me about the potential this approach has to transform their lives.

My original diet companions have also been reporting on their progress. Andrew and his office colleagues have incredible willpower:

> *Before Christmas, we had a box of chocolates given to us as a gift – on a diet day of course! We all speculated about scoffing the lot the next day – but guess what, none of use fancied them the next day! That indeed seems to be a theme – our overall appetite for eating more than we need has diminished. Most people I speak to are intrigued and usually think I'm on a food restricted diet until I explain more. I have to say I'm a bit of an evangelist, so I am pretty good at converting people – even some real sceptics.*

Like me, Tina is loving the health effects:

I think our emotional and mental wellbeing improves a lot on less food. I feel much more positive and clear headed if that makes sense. A bit like walking out on an early crisp cold morning and feeling really alive :). I guess that's the sharpness you mentioned. I used to take two lots of blood pressure tablets, but since losing weight my blood pressure dropped dramatically. I only discovered it because I started getting heart palpitations and went to my doc. He took my blood pressure, then told me to stand up. As I did he actually went 'whoa!'. My blood pressure dropped very low. After monitoring it and seeing how low it had become, he took me off the medication and for the first time in about twenty years, I'm medication free! My friends and family all think it's a great diet too. In fact both my sister in laws, my husband's niece and one of my friends have joined your group because they think I look great!

And Linda has been reaping the benefits too:

My mother had her six monthly family day just after Christmas and my nephew, who I hadn't seen for six months, commented, 'Good grief Linda, where's the rest of you gone?'! My only 'problem' is that having eaten low calorie foods for most of my life it's hard to eat anything like 'normal' calories on my 'feasting' days, so will often eat a couple of biscuits or have a glass of wine to make up the calories!

Scientists are busy continuing research into intermittent fasting and I'll be posting updates on www.the5-2dietbook.com – but I thought I'd end with the answers to the questions people have asked me recently.

Be honest – have you considered giving up this diet?

Not once. With pretty much every other diet I've undertaken, I've already given up by month four. On this one, I might have the odd day when circumstances change – I fancy going out to celebrate something, or a friend calls out of the blue. But there's no beating myself up – I simply switch the Fast Day to tomorrow. This isn't all or nothing – it's about a small but permanent change.

Will you abandon 5:2 once you reach the target?

No. I'm just two pounds away now and I like the idea of reducing to a fast one day a week, as a kind of 'check in' on portion size and for the health benefits. I'll also keep weighing myself once a week, because it's a good way to avoid the weight 'creeping' back on. Though I hope the changes to my appetite will also work in my favour there too.

Is this just another diet craze that will be forgotten by next Christmas?

My opinion – shared by many others – is that this really is different. It's not about cutting out entire food groups, or eating strange foods dreamed up by the diet industry. For me, it's about people who are overwhelmed by choice and the availability of food being helped to make better decisions. The natural appetite control, the flexibility, the health benefits and the all-round sustainability of it make it different.

Plus, it's a 'craze' that happens to have been around a very, very long time – from the unavoidable and frankly scary fast/feast lifestyle of early man, to the instructions to fast contained in so many religions. A respite or retreat from excess is something that has worked for humanity for many centuries. In the twentieth century, those who could, turned their back on the feeling of hunger, but now I've rediscovered what appetite and food mean to me.

A sense of perspective

I'm writing this on the evening of a Fast Day when I've eaten only one main meal, with no hunger pangs or ill effects. It reminds me how lucky we are to be able to choose what and when we eat. Fasting has done much more than help me lose weight – it's helped me regain control over my eating habits and make me look forward to my next meal as one of the pleasures of life.

I really hope you've been inspired by the stories of the fantastic dieters who shared their struggles and their successes. If you'd like your 5:2 journey to continue after this book, join us. We're @the52diet on Twitter, at facebook.com/groups/the52diet or on the new website, www.the5-2dietbook.com, where you can join the forums, find recipes or download free tools to make life easier. You can also get in touch with me there, I'd love to hear from you.

Finally, if you've enjoyed this book, or would like to recommend it to others, I'd be so grateful if you'd think about leaving a review.

In the meantime, keep feasting, keep fasting and keep enjoying life! Somehow, it all tastes so much better these days...

Kate x